THE
FAT-FREE
JUNK
FOOD
COOKBOOK

·····

Also by the author

The Fat-Free Real Food Cookbook

THE FAT-FREE JUNK FOOD COOKBOOK

100 Recipes of Guilt-Free Decadence

J. KEVIN WOLFE

Foreword by Lilias Folan

CROWN TRADE PAPERBACKS   NEW YORK

Published by Crown Trade Paperbacks, 201 East 50th Street, New York, New York 10022. Member of the Crown Publishing Group.

Random House, Inc. New York, Toronto, London, Sydney, Auckland

http://www.randomhouse.com/

Crown Trade Paperbacks and colophon are trademarks of Crown Publishers, Inc.

Originally published in different form by Im Press in 1993. Copyright © 1993 by J. Kevin Wolfe.

Printed in the United States of America

Library of Congress Cataloging-in-Publication Data
    The fat-free junk food cookbook: 100 recipes of guilt-free decadence/ by J. Kevin Wolfe.
        p.   cm.
    Includes index.
    1. Cookery.   2. Low-fat diet—Recipes.   3. Convenience foods.   I. Title.
    TX652.W64   1997
641.5—dc20   96-22315
        CIP

ISBN 0-517-88726-6

10 9 8 7 6 5 4 3 2 1

Updated Edition

*To my father, James E. Wolfe: The great kitchen
alchemist who taught me that no good recipe
should ever be left alone.*

C O N T E N T S

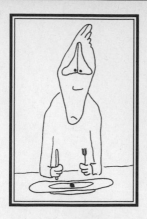

Acknowledgments 9
Foreword by Lilias Folan 11
Introduction 13

ACKNOWLEDGMENTS

Thanks to: Mom for cleaning up all those years, Marina for cleaning up all these years, Tristan and Melissa the top-notch Guinea pigs, James D. Vice the fudge architect, Aunt Helen Shigley and Mrs. Lottie Scott for the recipes, Dan Carraco for finding civilization that the "Weekly World News" missed, Catherine Brohaugh for making sense of the following, Bill Brohaugh for the road map, and Mike Martin for tech-support. Special thanks to two of the unsung avatars of cooking: Ed Espe Brown and Leah I. Swartz. Books can never replace teachers. But books by good teachers are the best substitute.

FOREWORD

My dad was a great cook. Some of my fondest memories of my father are of him wildly cooking up a storm in our small kitchen when I was fourteen years old. Pots boiling, steam rising, lots of father–daughter communication. I was the parsley chopper. He gave the orders. I was the refrigerator runner. He poured on the heavy cream and butter.

Those days of heavy cream and butter are gone. Yes, I miss their taste. But when a book like *The Fat-Free Junk Food Cookbook* comes along, it makes the transition fun and easy. It reeducates the taste buds deliciously. And it slims the waist almost effortlessly. My family and I are enjoying these recipes, and you will too.

Men are great cooks, don't you agree?

Lilias Folan

INTRODUCTION

My Fight with Fat

In April 1993 I was pushing two hundred pounds. For a five-foot seven-inch human, that's long past the point when you're embarrassed to be seen at the pool.

I had seen my hero, and the world's most followed yogi, Lilias Folan, on TV still looking incredibly fit as I ballooned. I knew I had to do something.

So I went on a low-fat diet. And I discovered there was nothing good left to eat. I wanted brownies, cookies, and ice cream, but even one serving of any of these treats would get me pulled over by the pudge police for exceeding my twenty-five-gram-a-day fat limit.

So I started working on fat-free junk food. I looked for ways of improving existing no-fat recipes. I found fat placebos for my favorite recipes. I started from scratch and created new recipes.

No fat. No guilt. No gain. As a matter of fact, during the initial experimentation for this book between April and July 1993, I lost thirty-three pounds.

I didn't even count calories. My portions of low-fat food were unrestricted. I could eat all the red beans and rice I wanted. If I craved an extra helping of fat-free jam cake for dessert, fine. (I said, "an extra helping," not "the whole cake"!)

I lost weight, but more importantly I've kept it off, even through the dreaded winter holidays. Here are the best of the fat-free recipes that I, and my family, have come to love. I hope you find them as gooey, juicy, tasty, and helpful as I do. Many take less than thirty minutes to prepare and cook. The ☕ tells you the amount of precooking preparation time for each recipe. The 🍲 shows you the total time the recipe takes, start to finish, including cooking time.

The Fat-Free Fine Print

The words "fat-free" are flying around more these days than UFOs over Graceland. Here's the real truth. "Fat-free" does not mean a food contains absolutely no fat: By FDA guidelines "fat-free" means that a serving of food contains one-half gram of fat or less.

This can be misleading. Here's an example: A large snack food company is peddling fat-free devil's food cookies that contain just under one-half gram of fat per cookie. On the box, a serving is listed as one cookie. People were once willing to hijack this company's trucks to get these cookies.

A smaller company is producing the same cookie at the same factory with a slightly altered recipe. They have been doing so for years. Each of their cookies also contains just under one-half gram of fat. On the back of their box, a serving is listed as two cookies. So per-serving fat content is listed as one gram. Nobody buys cookie B. Yet both brands of cookies have virtually the same fat content. The difference? The big company has a better marketing department.

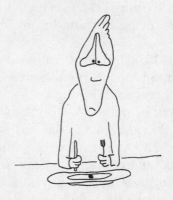

Very few things are truly fat-free. Flour has one gram of fat per cup. Skim milk has one-half gram of fat per cup. Even vegetables contain trace amounts of fat. That being said, all the recipes in this book have one-half gram of fat or less per serving. I've kept the serving sizes as generous as possible.

The fat content of the recipes in this book was estimated by using the most current fat-content information from the manufacturers of the ingredients used. Fat content added in the preparation, by cooking spray, for example, and by the use of cornmeal on cooking surfaces, was also factored in. To keep these recipes fat-free, please use the ingredients listed, in the portions listed. There will always be slight fat-content variations in ingredients from manufacturer to manufacturer and from batch to batch. (For more, see "Reading the Label" on page 86.)

The serving size has been calculated to contain less than one-half gram of fat. If you increase the serving size, your portion will no longer be fat-free. However, even if you increase your portion by six, it will still be low-fat according to FDA guidelines.

A Lower-Fat Life

Some tips for reducing fat:

▶ If you must fry, fry with vegetable oil cooking spray or with ¼ teaspoon of oil rubbed on your skillet before heating.

▶ If fat-free products like cream cheese, sour cream, and mayo don't appeal to you, try mixing ¼ cup of the real thing with ¾ cup of the fat-free.

▶ Find a fat-free salad dressing you like and carry it with you at all times.

▶ If fat-free cheeses aren't for you, try cheeses that are high in flavor but naturally lower in fat, such as feta and Parmesan.

▶ Keep lots of low-fat snacks on hand for tempting moments. Fruit, carrots, and celery are healthy. Try mixing tiny pretzels and miniature marshmallows. It sounds like an odd combo but it's really satisfying. It's salty, sweet, chewy, and crunchy at the same time.

▶ Find veggies you like and eat lots of them. The more healthy vegetables you eat, the less you'll consume of the fattening part of the meal.

▶ Eat because you're hungry, not because you feel a compulsion. Always give yourself the freedom to eat as much low-fat food as you want. But ask yourself, "Am I truly hungry for this?" If you aren't, don't eat it, but if you are, eat and *enjoy*.

▶ When eating out, ask how your food is prepared. Many foods that start out low in fat are then prepared with a lot of fat. Find out exactly what you're getting. Many restaurants will be happy to accommodate you if you ask that your food be prepared using as little fat as possible.

▶ Count your fat grams. Learn the fat content of foods in your diet and you'll soon be aware of how many fat grams you've eaten that day without having to think about it.

▶ Eat protein and carbohydrates together. The combination fills you up much better than protein or carbohydrates alone. That's why a fat-free cheese sandwich seems more satisfying than a fat-free cookie.

1

▼

Concession Stand Snacks

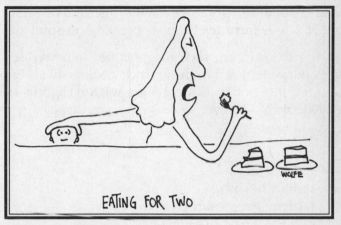

EATING FOR TWO

- ▶ **I SWEAR THEY'RE FAT-FREE FRENCH FRIES**
- ▶ **CRISPY CRISPIX MIX**
- ▶ **HONEY MUSTARD CHEX**
- ▶ **CRISPY BARBECUE SNACKS**
- ▶ **CHILI CHEESE CRUNCHES**
- ▶ **CRUNCHY CARAMEL CORN**
- ▶ **SCORCHING NACHOS**
- ▶ **LAGER CHEESE LITE**

I Swear They're Fat-Free French Fries

▼▼▼▼▼▼▼

Finally! Fat-free fries that taste like fries! Crisp outside, tender and moist inside.

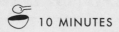 10 MINUTES  20 MINUTES

MAKES 2 SERVINGS.

Bake **3 medium potatoes** in the microwave until tender (about **3 to 4 minutes** each, depending on spud size).

Leaving the skin on, slice the potatoes into wedges. Place them skin-side down on a nonstick cookie sheet. Brush the meat of the potato with **1 egg white** (lightly beaten). Sprinkle with whatever spice strikes your fancy:

> **salt**
> **pepper**
> **Cajun spices**
> **Italian herbs**
> **fat-free Parmesan cheese**
> **Old Bay Seasoning**
> **taco seasoning**
> (let your imagination take over)

Broil in the oven about **10 minutes,** until golden brown.

Dip in:

> **ketchup**
> **barbecue sauce**
> **fat-free mayonnaise**
> **fat-free ranch dressing**
> **taco sauce**
> **vinegar**
> (let your imagination take over again)

CRISPY CRISPIX MIX

▼▼▼▼▼▼▼

Most crispy snacks like potato chips or corn chips contain ten grams of fat per ounce. But one cup of this snack is fat-free. Crispix, Chex, even Cheerios cereal can be used. If you want to get fancy, substitute an equal amount of fat-free bagel chips, fat-free melba toast chips, or fat-free pretzels for the cereal.

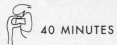 10 MINUTES 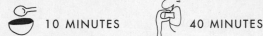 40 MINUTES

MAKES THREE 1-CUP SERVINGS.

Preheat oven to **250°F.**

In a large bowl, combine the following:

> **1 tablespoon Worcestershire sauce**
> **1 teaspoon onion powder**
> **1 teaspoon garlic powder**
> **1½ teaspoons salt**
> **1½ teaspoons sugar**
> **3 tablespoons water**

Mix in:

> **3 cups Crispix**

Turn GENTLY with a fork until the cereal is covered with sauce. Spread onto nonstick cookie sheets. Keep the cereal one layer thick and keep the sides of the snacks from touching.

Bake for **20 minutes.**

Let cool 15 minutes before removing from cookie sheets.

For best results, store sealed.

MICROWAVE: Cook on high for 5 minutes, turning every 30 seconds. Keep the snacks to the edges of the pan. They have a tendency to catch fire when in the middle.

CONCESSION STAND SNACKS

19

HONEY MUSTARD CHEX

▼▼▼▼▼▼▼

Take these to work to munch on. It's best not to leave them out on your desk if you want to eat some yourself.

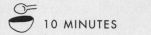 10 MINUTES   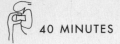 40 MINUTES

MAKES THREE 1-CUP SERVINGS.

Preheat oven to **250°F.**

In a medium bowl, mix:

> **¼ cup Dijon mustard**
> **2 tablespoons honey**
> **1 tablespoon dry mustard**
> **1½ teaspoons onion powder**

Stir well. Add:

> **3 cups Chex**

Turn GENTLY with a fork until the cereal is covered with sauce.

Spread onto nonstick cookie sheets. Keep the cereal one layer thick and don't let the sides of the snacks touch each other.

Bake for **20 minutes.**

Let cool 15 minutes before removing from cookie sheets.

Store in sealed container.

MICROWAVE: Cook on high for 5 minutes, turning every 30 seconds. Place the snacks toward the edges of the dish to keep them from burning.

CRISPY BARBECUE SNACKS

▼▼▼▼▼▼▼

Barbecue sauce gives these snacks great flavor. They're a terrific complement to sandwiches.

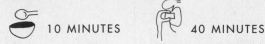 10 MINUTES   40 MINUTES

MAKES THREE 1-CUP SERVINGS.

Preheat oven to **250°F.**

In a large bowl, mix:

⅓ cup barbecue sauce
1 tablespoon salt
½ teaspoon chili powder

With a fork, GENTLY turn in:

3 cups Crispix

Place snacks side by side, but not touching, on nonstick cookie sheets.

Bake for **20 minutes.**

Let cool 15 minutes before removing from pan.

Store sealed.

MICROWAVE: Cook on high for 5 minutes, turning every 30 seconds. Keep the snacks toward the edge of the pan. They may burn if left in the middle.

VARIATION: For hotter, smokier snacks, add 1 teaspoon cayenne pepper and ½ teaspoon Liquid Smoke.

CHILI CHEESE CRUNCHES

▼▼▼▼▼▼▼

Yogurt is what gives these snacks a hint of cheese flavor. They're not at all sweet, and they're a perfect match with colas and lunch.

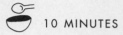 10 MINUTES   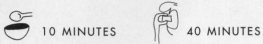 40 MINUTES

MAKES THREE 1-CUP SERVINGS.

Preheat oven to **250°F.**

In a large bowl, mix:

> **⅔ cup plain fat-free yogurt**
> **1½ teaspoons salt**
> **2 tablespoons ground coriander**
> **⅓ cup chili powder**
> **2 tablespoons sugar**
> **3 tablespoons garlic powder**
> **1 teaspoon black pepper**

With a fork, GENTLY turn in:

3 cups cereal like Chex (any kind) until covered.

Place snacks side by side, but not touching, on nonstick cookie sheets.

Bake for **20 minutes.**

Let cool 15 minutes and remove.

MICROWAVE: Cook on high for 5 minutes, turning every 30 seconds. Keep the snacks toward the edge of the pan. They might burn if left in the center.

CRUNCHY CARAMEL CORN

▼▼▼▼▼▼▼

We think popcorn is a healthy snack, but that's not always the case. When corn is air-popped, it's fat-free. However, some makers of caramel corn pop the corn in oil and then add large quantities of butter to the caramel coating. This means that commercial caramel corn may contain six or more grams of fat in a cupful. This recipe, on the other hand, is fat-free.

25 MINUTES

MAKES FOUR 1-CUP SERVINGS.

Place **4 cups hot air-popped popcorn** in a large bowl that's been lightly sprayed with vegetable oil cooking spray. Set aside. In a medium saucepan, mix:

½ cup brown sugar
2 tablespoons buttermilk
¼ teaspoon salt

Cook over medium heat. Drop a few drips of the liquid into a cup of cold water. The glaze is ready when these drops form tiny balls that can be picked up with your fingers.

Pour the glaze over the popcorn and stir IMMEDIATELY. The caramel corn can be molded into balls or eaten loose. When it's cool enough to touch, it's ready to eat.

WHERE DO THEY FIND THESE PEOPLE WHO MAKE THESE DIET CLAIMS?

THE LUSCIOUS LUST DIET PLAN: "Not only did I lose the weight, but the diet increased my sex drive so much I became a bigamist."

THE MELTING MOVEMENT TANNING BUTTER DIET: "The fat not only melted away, but when it became liquid I rubbed it on for this perfect golden tan."

Scorching Nachos

▾ ▾ ▾ ▾ ▾ ▾ ▾

Nachos no longer need to be fattening. Try this at your next informal gathering.

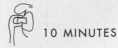 10 MINUTES

MAKES SEVEN 1-OUNCE SERVINGS.

In a microwave-safe bowl, mix:

6 ounces shredded fat-free cheddar cheese
3 tablespoons fat-free salsa (most are, but check
  the package)
1 tablespoon diced onion

Set microwave for **3 minutes** on high. Take out and stir mixture in bowl every 30 seconds. If you don't you'll wind up with a large yellow hockey puck.

Pour onto:

Baked low-fat tortilla chips topped with **jalapeños, onions,** and **fat-free refried beans.**

Lager Cheese Lite

▾ ▾ ▾ ▾ ▾ ▾ ▾

If you're not a beer drinker, don't worry. This beer cheese has very little beer in it. A few tablespoons give it some moisture.

For parties, serve it with an unsliced loaf of white or rye bread. Hollow out the bread as you would a jack-o'-lantern (don't cut eyes or a mouth, though). Spoon the beer cheese into the bread bowl. Surround the bowl with 1½-inch bread cubes for dipping.

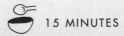 15 MINUTES

MAKES SIXTEEN 1-OUNCE SERVINGS.

In a food processor, blend the following:

6 ounces fat-free cottage cheese
6 ounces fat-free cheddar cheese
a pinch garlic powder
2 tablespoons chopped onion
2 tablespoons fat-free salsa
**enough beer to get it moving in the food
processor** (it's supposed to be thick, so don't use
too much beer or you'll get soup)

Process until smooth. Chill at least 3 hours before serving.

DEALING WITH THE HOLIDAYS

During the winter holiday months the average person puts on ten pounds.

It starts innocently enough. A big meal at Thanksgiving. Then comes holiday shopping. You don't have time to fix anything, so you grab your meals at the mall. Then come the holiday parties. You always find yourself dropping by twice as many as you had planned. And there's eggnog and that favorite dessert you just had to have a little bite of, maybe two. Okay, maybe three . . . Hey, where'd that slice on my plate go?

Then come holiday dinners. Then post-holiday dinners to get rid of the leftovers. Then New Year's parties. Then it's the middle of January, and too late to make a resolution. May as well start that diet in the spring when it's warm enough to exercise. Pass the Oreos, would you?

We've all been through it. But this year you can do something different: Change your holiday eating habits and you won't have those extra pounds to lose next year.

At your house, YOU control what goes on the table. Make sure there are plenty of vegetables and some fat-free bread (page 70). If you're going to someone else's house, volunteer to take some sinless Banana Eggnog (pages 132–133) or Hot Spiced Cider (page 133). Take a gooey dessert. No one needs to know it's fat-free. Make the effort. Your bathroom scale will thank you, come January.

2

Fast Food

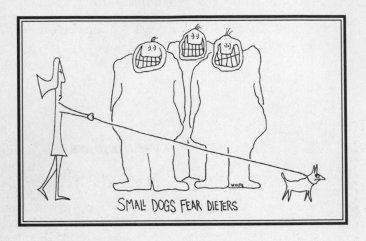

SMALL DOGS FEAR DIETERS

- ▶ WORLD'S THINNEST PIZZA CRUST
- ▶ K-K-KRISPY PIZZA CRUST
- ▶ GOLDEN FLATBREAD
- ▶ ZINGY PIZZA SAUCE
- ▶ PIZZA BLANCA SAUCE
- ▶ THE WHOLE TOMATO SAUCE

- ▶ "THEY SURE DON'T TASTE LIKE" VEGEBURGERS

- ▶ FAT-FREE DRIPPIN' BURGERS

- ▶ STINGING WING SAUCE

- ▶ TACOS

- ▶ EASY CHEESY FONDUE

Pizza can be a fat-free meal. However, frozen pizza and restaurant pizza can contain up to fifteen grams of fat per slice. The problem is mostly in the cheese and topping. Here you'll find three great fat-free pizza crusts and sauces—the building blocks. Then try the following great-tasting, guilt-less toppings, with or without fat-free cheese. (If you place fat-free cheese under the sauce and other ingredients, it will actually melt and not turn into dried leather.)

Guiltless toppings: onions, green bell peppers, red bell peppers, ¼ cup jalapeño peppers, banana peppers, mush-rooms, nonmarinated artichoke hearts, 1 teaspoon imitation bacon bits, broccoli, spinach, pineapple.

WORLD'S THINNEST PIZZA CRUST
▼▼▼▼▼▼▼

This recipe is for those who like a crispy thin pizza crust. It can be made as thin as a cracker. The thinner it is, the bet-ter the taste. Break one into large pieces to eat with soup, dip, or spreads.

40 MINUTES

MAKES 6 CRUSTS.

Put a cast-iron skillet on a burner and set the heat to high.

In a medium metal or glass bowl, mix:

> **1½ cups flour**
> **¼ teaspoon salt**
> **1 teaspoon Italian seasoning** (oregano, thyme, sage, rosemary, and basil)
> **½ cup water**

Using a fork, knead the dough for 3 minutes.

Pull off a piece of dough the size of a golf ball. Roll it out using a rolling pin. Use as much flour as is necessary to keep the dough from sticking to the pin or the working surface. When it's rolled to the thickness of a burrito, lay it flat in the hot skillet.

Cook **30 seconds to 2 minutes** on each side (depending how brown you want the crust).

Add pizza sauce (pages 31–32), no-fat cheese, or whatever toppings you wish. Pop under the broiler or in the oven at 350°F. for **10 minutes.**

Note: These crusts can be stored for later use, but they're so crispy that they'll pick up moisture from the air no matter what you put them in. A sealed tin is best. They can be crisped up by popping them in the oven at 325°F. for a few minutes.

K-K-KRISPY PIZZA CRUST

▼ ▼ ▼ ▼ ▼ ▼ ▼

This recipe for traditional pizza crust takes some time. You have to let the dough go through two risings. Using the "knead only" or "manual" cycle, this recipe works very well in a bread machine.

 20 MINUTES   1 HOUR 20 MINUTES

MAKES ONE 14-INCH CRUST.

In a medium bowl, dissolve:

> **2 teaspoons yeast**
> **1 teaspoon sugar**

in

> **½ cup warm water**

Mix in:

> **½ teaspoon salt**
> **1¼ cups flour**

Knead in more flour until the dough is tacky, but no longer sticks to your hands (3 to 5 minutes).

Cover and let rise in a warm place for **30 minutes.**

Preheat oven to **425°F.**

On a floured work surface, punch down the dough and roll out with a floured rolling pin until it's large enough to cover your pizza pan.

Sprinkle **1 teaspoon cornmeal** over a pizza pan. Place the dough in the pan. Top with **fat-free mozzarella cheese, pizza sauce** (pages 31–32), and lots of **vegetables.** Remember: Most vegetables are fat-free, so pile them on.

Bake for **20 to 25 minutes,** until the crust is starting to brown a little underneath.

BREAD MACHINE OPTION: Place the yeast in one corner of the machine's mixing bowl. Add salt, flour, and water. Set machine to "manual" or "knead only." Push START. When the dough is ready, roll out. Sprinkle 1 teaspoon cornmeal on a pizza pan. Place dough in the pan. Top and bake.

GOLDEN FLATBREAD
▼▼▼▼▼▼▼

Golden Flatbread is a beautiful, round, flat loaf. It looks kind of like a tanned mutant pita. But it's light and full of tiny air pockets, which give it a creamy texture. The golden color makes it a guest-worthy sight.

It can be sliced into wedges and eaten with soups or salads. It can be used as a deep-dish pizza crust or fruit pizza base (see pages 29–30). Or it can be sliced flat to make a giant stuffed sandwich.

 50 MINUTES   2 HOURS 10 MINUTES

MAKES 3 LOAVES; EACH LOAF SERVES 4.

Make **Ultralight Pastry Dough** (pages 66–67) through the second rise.

Preheat oven to **350°F.**

Divide dough into 3 equal balls. On a floured surface, roll out each ball into a 14-inch circle, ¼ inch thick.

Sprinkle **1 teaspoon cornmeal** on each of 3 cookie sheets. Lay one circle of dough on each sheet. Brush with **egg wash** (1 egg white mixed with 2 tablespoons skim milk).

Let rise for **20 minutes.**

Bake for **15 to 20 minutes,** until the tops are golden brown. Cool on a wire rack. Store in a sealed container.

VARIATION: For deep-dish pizza, after the final rising of the Ultralight Pastry Dough, top with The Whole Tomato Sauce (pages 32–33) and toppings and bake for 20 to 25 minutes. As soon as you pull it out of the oven, top with fat-free mozzarella.

ZINGY PIZZA SAUCE

▼ ▼ ▼ ▼ ▼ ▼

A serving of most canned pizza sauce is fat-free or low-fat. If you don't have any canned sauce around, this is easy to make and keeps well in the fridge.

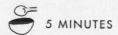 5 MINUTES

MAKES THREE ½-CUP SERVINGS.

In a small bowl, mix:

  1 8-ounce can tomato sauce
  ½ 6-ounce can tomato paste
  1 teaspoon garlic powder
  1 tablespoon Italian seasoning (oregano, thyme, sage, rosemary, and basil)

Spread over pizza dough.

Pizza Blanca Sauce

▼▼▼▼▼▼▼

For some people, a pizza IS cheese. Use this sauce instead of a red sauce to satisfy that cheese monkey on your back.

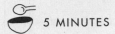 5 MINUTES

MAKES TWO ¼-CUP SERVINGS.

In a small bowl, mix:

> **½ cup fat-free ricotta cheese**
> **½ teaspoon salt**
> **2 finely minced garlic cloves**

Spread over pizza dough.

VARIATION: Top with raw spinach and cooked broccoli.

The Whole Tomato Sauce

▼▼▼▼▼▼▼

Pizza sauce is no longer spaghetti sauce with sugar in it. This version has a tangy taste. You can use fresh tomatoes, but they don't get tender enough. Most pizza places use canned, frozen, or rehydrated Roma tomatoes.

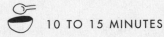 10 TO 15 MINUTES

MAKES TWO ½-CUP SERVINGS.

Coarsely chop:

> **8 ounces drained canned whole tomatoes**

Place the chopped tomatoes in a colander for **5 minutes** to drain off any excess liquid.

In a small bowl, mix:

2 minced garlic cloves
1 tablespoon Italian seasoning (oregano, thyme, sage, rosemary, and basil)

Spread over pizza.

Slather it on. The whole batch is fat-free.

"THEY SURE DON'T TASTE LIKE" VEGEBURGERS

▼▼▼▼▼▼▼

Vegeburgers have gotten a bad rap, because they're always being compared to hamburgers. They're not for everyone, but they're an excellent alternative for those bold enough to try them. The beans and egg whites provide enough protein to satisfy the appetite, and they're flavorful and hearty enough for meat lovers.

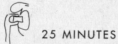

25 MINUTES

MAKES 3 OR 4 BURGERS.

In a medium bowl, mix the following:

⅔ cup black beans (mashed)
1½ cups fat-free bread crumbs (store-bought, or see page 70)
2 tablespoons steak sauce
½ teaspoon garlic powder
1 egg white
½ teaspoon salt (or seasoning salt)

Shape into 3 or 4 patties. Fry until firm in a skillet lightly coated with vegetable oil cooking spray. (Once fried, these burgers can be frozen, then reheated and crisped in the toaster.)

Someone did some research a few years back that determined that Americans didn't want low-fat hot dogs. If they were going to down a dog, they wanted all the fat. But if you put tons of trimmings on a low-fat hot dog, these same people probably wouldn't be able to tell the difference.

Use low-fat buns and low-fat dogs and top with the following fat-free items: ketchup, mustard, onions, pickle relish, sauerkraut, fat-free cheddar cheese, fat-free sharp cheese.

Make taco dogs using fat-free taco filling (page 36), onions, salsa, and fat-free cheddar cheese.

FAT-FREE DRIPPIN' BURGERS

▼▼▼▼▼▼▼

Burgers are usually the first thing people cut out when they go on a diet. If prepared properly, they can be very low in fat. These burgers are flavorful and can be skillet-fried or grilled. The Worcestershire sauce not only adds flavor, but also gives the burgers a darker, more beef-like color.

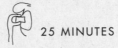 25 MINUTES

MAKES 3 BURGERS.

Put the following ingredients in a food processor:

> **4 ounces 99% fat-free turkey breast cutlets**
> **1 egg white**
> **2 tablespoons steak sauce**
> **2 slices fat-free bread**
> **½ teaspoon garlic powder**
> **½ teaspoon salt**
> **1 teaspoon Worcestershire sauce**

Blend until the consistency of raw hamburger. Form into 3 patties. Fry in a skillet, or grill. (Cooked patties can also be frozen and thawed and then reheated.)

It's best not to overcook these burgers as they have very little fat in them to keep them juicy. Top with **fat-free cheese,** or, for a low-fat bacon and cheese burger, sprinkle the cheese with **imitation bacon bits.**

VARIATION: Substitute seasoning salt for the steak sauce or Worcestershire. Substitute ¼ cup fat-free cracker crumbs for the bread.

STINGING WING SAUCE

▼▼▼▼▼▼

Authentic Buffalo Wing sauce is made from two ingredients in equal parts: cayenne pepper sauce and butter. That gives it about eight grams of fat per tablespoon. On the other hand, one tablespoon of this sauce is fat-free. The vinegar preserves this sauce well, so refrigeration is not necessary.

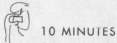 10 MINUTES

MAKES FIVE 1-TABLESPOON SERVINGS OF SAUCE.

Mix the following in a small bowl:

¼ cup cayenne pepper sauce (Louisiana Hot, Durkee Red Hot)
1 teaspoon dry mustard
1 tablespoon vinegar

Note: Authentic Buffalo Wings are not batter-fried. That's a good thing, because one chicken wing alone contains about two grams of fat. Grill the wings, basting with the sauce. They'll be a little wetter if you brush on the sauce afterward. Serve with **celery** and **fat-free blue cheese dressing.** This quells the lingering heat of the wings.

TACOS

▼▼▼▼▼▼▼

Taco filling is usually made with the fattiest ground beef available. The grease is used in combination with flour to "bind" the meat. However, you can make it deliciously fat-free.

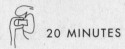 20 MINUTES

MAKES ENOUGH FAT-FREE FILLING FOR 4 OR 5 TACOS.

In a food processor, process **8 ounces 99% fat-free turkey breast cutlets** until they're the size of BBs.

Cook in a skillet over medium heat until the meat turns white. Add:

> ½ **teaspoon salt**
> **1 tablespoon chili powder**
> **1 tablespoon flour**
> ½ **teaspoon garlic powder**

Continue cooking until the meat is bound together.

Place into a **taco shell** (3 grams of fat) or in a **fat-free burrito shell** or **flour tortilla.**

Top with:

> **lettuce or spinach** (shredded)
> **onions**
> **tomatoes**
> **taco sauce**
> **fat-free cheddar cheese**

EASY CHEESY FONDUE

▼▼▼▼▼▼▼

Cheese fondue is a good intimate party food for four to six people. This recipe uses fat-free mozzarella cheese, which most people never acquire a taste for in its unaltered state. But heat it with a little white wine and garlic and it becomes quite palatable. *For dessert, heat up some Hot Fudgy Milk Chocolate Sauce (page 113) for chocolate fondue.*

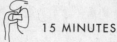 15 MINUTES

MAKES TWELVE 1-OUNCE SERVINGS.

In a warm fondue pot, mix:

12 ounces fat-free mozzarella cheese
3 tablespoons white wine
½ teaspoon finely minced garlic

Stir constantly until the cheese melts. Dip **fat-free bread cubes** in the cheese sauce. Keep it warm or it will harden.

MICROWAVE: Put the cheese, wine, and garlic in a microwave-safe bowl. Cook on high for 3 minutes. Remove every 30 seconds and stir, or you'll wind up with baked French rubber.

SANDWICH SUGGESTIONS

Sandwiches can be as high in fat or as low in fat as you wish. Low-fat bread is available in white, wheat, and rye.

Fishwiches: Grilled fish (such as cod, grouper, or haddock), fat-free sharp American cheese, and low-fat tartar sauce

Club sandwiches: Low-fat turkey and beef, lettuce, fat-free mayo

Reuben sandwiches: Low-fat rye, low-fat corned beef, sauerkraut, fat-free Swiss or mozzarella cheese, Dijon mustard

Chicken sandwiches: Grilled chicken breast, fat-free ranch dressing, fat-free sharp American cheese, lettuce

3

Brunch: The Mid-Morning Pigout

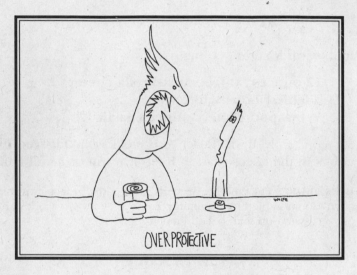

OVERPROTECTIVE

- ▶ **WICKED CINNAMON ROLLS**
- ▶ **SWEET CHEESE PUFFS**
- ▶ **SKINNY CINNAMON TOAST**
- ▶ **LA TOAST FRANÇAISE**
- ▶ **FRUIT JUICE FLAPJACKS**
- ▶ **AIRY BUTTERMILK PANCAKES**

- ▶ **1-2-3-4-5 Spicebread**

- ▶ **1-2-3-4-5 Citrus Bread**

- ▶ **1-2-3-4-5 Cinnamon Bread**

- ▶ **Ultra-Crunch Granola**

- ▶ **Shaker Bread Pudding with Oozing Caramel Sauce**

WICKED CINNAMON ROLLS

▼▼▼▼▼▼▼

These monstrous cinnamon rolls, oozing with brown sugar and cinnamon, nearly fall under the weight of their thick frosting. They go beyond sinful; they're nearly satanic. But they're still fat-free, so there's no need to go to confession.

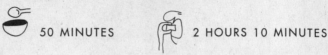

50 MINUTES   2 HOURS 10 MINUTES

MAKES 7 BIG ROLLS.

Make **Ultralight Pastry Dough** (pages 66–67) through the second rise.

Sprinkle flour onto a work surface. Place the dough on top. Sprinkle enough flour on the dough to keep it from sticking to your rolling pin. Roll the dough flat until it's about ¼ inch thick. Work the corners with the rolling pin and try to get a rectangular shape rather than a circle.

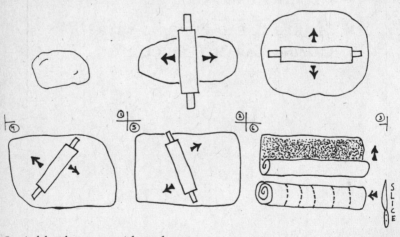

Sprinkle the top with at least:

1 cup brown sugar
2 tablespoons ground cinnamon (don't be stingy: neither contains fat)

Gently roll dough rectangle into a log from the long side. Slice into sections 2 inches thick. Place on a nonstick rimmed cookie sheet. (The more brown sugar you use, the more it oozes out the bottom of the rolls.)

Preheat oven to **375°F.**

Brush rolls with an egg wash made of:

> **1 egg white**
> **1 tablespoon skim milk**

Let rise for **20 minutes.**

Bake for **20 minutes,** until the tops are light golden brown. Remove immediately from the pan. Ice heavily. (Recipe follows.)

Note: You can also freeze the rolls before baking. Place unbaked rolls in a foil lasagne pan. Cover tightly with foil lid. They can then be baked straight from the freezer. When ready to make, remove lid and bake for 25 minutes at 375°F.

► **THE FROSTING THAT** ◄
MOVES LIKE A SLOTH

MAKES ½ CUP.

Pour **1⅓ cups powdered sugar** into a small bowl.

Boil **2 tablespoons skim milk.** Pour over sugar and stir until smooth.

Add **1 teaspoon vanilla extract.** Stir until well mixed. Spoon onto cinnamon rolls. The whole batch of frosting is fat-free.

VARIATION: Cold lemon juice can be used in place of the milk for a frosting that's more tangy.

SWEET CHEESE PUFFS

▼ ▼ ▼ ▼ ▼ ▼ ▼

Cheese danishes contain up to ten grams of fat per serving. These sweet cheese puffs, on the other hand, are fat-free.

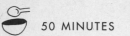 50 MINUTES   2 HOURS 10 MINUTES

MAKES 12 PUFFS.

Make **Ultralight Pastry Dough** (pages 66–67) through the second rise.

Place flour on a work surface. Place dough on top, and sprinkle with enough flour to keep it from sticking to your rolling pin.

Roll out until it's ¾ inch thick. Cut into squares 2½ by 2½ inches. Place squares into the cups of a 12-cup nonstick muffin tin. Gently press into bottom of each cup.

Brush the tops with **egg wash** (1 egg white mixed with 2 tablespoons skim milk).

Let rise for **20 minutes.**

While dough is rising, in a small bowl, mix:

> **1 cup fat-free ricotta cheese**
> **¼ cup sugar**
> **1 teaspoon vanilla extract**

After puffs have risen, use your finger to firmly push down the center of each cup. Place **1 heaping teaspoon cheese mixture** into each depression.

Bake for **20 minutes.**

Remove immediately from tin. Serve warm.

SKINNY CINNAMON TOAST

▼ ▼ ▼ ▼ ▼ ▼ ▼

This cinnamon toast is spicy and heavy on the sugar. It's best when eaten right out of the oven.

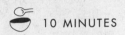 10 MINUTES   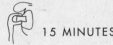 15 MINUTES

MAKES 6 SERVINGS.

Start with **6 slices fat-free bread** (store-bought, or see page 70).

Place on a nonstick cookie sheet. Spread with **fat-free margarine** or spray lightly with **I Can't Believe It's Not Butter spray.**

Liberally sprinkle **sugar** and **ground cinnamon** on top of margarine.

Place under broiler until the edges of the bread are brown.

THE FORTY-GRAM RULE

There's an equation floating around today that states: If you eat more than forty grams of fat a day, you gain weight; if you eat less than forty grams of fat a day, you lose weight.

There are other factors, but this rule seems to work for most people. So just how much food is forty grams of fat?

ON THE DOWNSIDE: It's 1½ Quarter Pounders with Cheese. It's 1½ Dove Bars. It's 1⅓ KFC Thighs.

ON THE UPSIDE: It's more than 2½ pounds of pretzels. It's more than a dozen bags of marshmallows. It's more than a grocery sack of hard candy. It's also lots and lots of fruit, vegetables, beans, and grains, but the junk food seems to grab more attention.

LA TOAST FRANÇAISE

▼ ▼ ▼ ▼ ▼ ▼ ▼

Loads of powdered sugar and rivers of syrup aren't what make French toast fattening. It's the egg yolks, the cream, and the oil that you fry it in. This version is more bourgeois than regular French toast, but it's still fat-free. The Cointreau liqueur gives it a mild, sweet orange flavor.

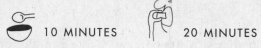 10 MINUTES   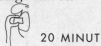 20 MINUTES

MAKES 6 SERVINGS.

Combine in a bowl:

> **4 ounces Egg Beaters**
> **2 tablespoons skim milk** (or fat-free Ice Cream, pages 110–11)
> **2 tablespoons Cointreau** (or any orange liqueur: Curaçao, Triple Sec, or Grand Marnier are all fine)
> **1 teaspoon ground cinnamon**
> **a pinch ground cloves** (and only a pinch)

Whip with a wire whisk until the batter gets foamy. You'll need **6 thick slices sweet white bread** (page 70), about 1 inch thick. (Any fat-free bread will do, but a light-white pastry bread is best.)

DIP both sides of the bread in the batter. Don't soak the bread, or your toast will get tough.

Cook over medium heat in a skillet that's been lightly coated with cooking spray. Turn when lightly browned.

Dust with powdered sugar and have some warm maple syrup ready.

Brunch Serving Suggestions

- ◆ Garnish with a few orange wedges.
- ◆ Serve with fresh sliced melon.
- ◆ Spoon some fat-free cottage cheese alongside the toast.

LOWER-FAT OMELETS

An egg yolk contains six grams of fat. That means that a three-egg omelet contains eighteen grams of fat, not including the oil you cook it in, the cheese, or the bacon. For lower-fat omelets:

Use cooking spray rather than oil in the pan.

Use Egg Beaters.

Use only one yolk and three egg whites.

Use grated fat-free cheese and imitation bacon bits.

Load your omelet with fat-free ingredients such as mushrooms, green bell peppers, and artichokes.

FRUIT JUICE FLAPJACKS

▼ ▼ ▼ ▼ ▼ ▼ ▼

Using fruit juice to moisten pancakes eliminates fat and gives them a sweet, refreshing taste. It also neatly gets in your juice quota without having to actually drink it.

The acid from the fruit juice activates the baking soda. You'll get lighter, fluffier cakes from higher-acid citrus juices. But most fruit juices have enough tartness to give you a satisfactory flapjack. Try orange juice, pineapple juice, apple cider, cranberry juice (with vitamin C added), kiwi, strawberry, or apricot nectar.

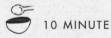 10 MINUTES 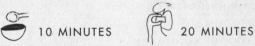 20 MINUTES

MAKES 2 DOZEN PANCAKES; 4 PANCAKES CONTAIN LESS THAN ONE-HALF GRAM OF FAT.

In a medium bowl, mix the following ingredients one at a time, stirring well after each addition:

3 egg whites
2 cups fruit juice
2 cups flour
½ teaspoon salt
1 teaspoon baking soda

With a large spoon, pour batter into a hot nonstick skillet that's been lightly sprayed with vegetable oil cooking spray. Flip when the bottoms start to brown. Serve immediately.

AIRY BUTTERMILK PANCAKES

▼ ▼ ▼ ▼ ▼ ▼ ▼

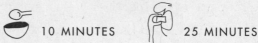 10 MINUTES   25 MINUTES

MAKES 2 DOZEN PANCAKES; ONE PANCAKE CONTAINS LESS THAN ONE-HALF GRAM OF FAT.

A pancake breakfast no longer needs to be high in fat. You can't use butter on top of these fat-free flapjacks, but you can use powdered sugar and maple syrup, which are both fat-free. (These pancakes are moist, so fat-free margarine is not necessary, but you can add it if you miss seeing something yellow on top.)

In a large bowl, beat:

3 egg whites until they start to get bubbly

Mix in the following ingredients one at a time. Blend well after each addition:

2½ cups buttermilk
½ teaspoon salt
1 teaspoon baking soda
2 cups flour

Pour the batter into a hot nonstick skillet that's been lightly sprayed with vegetable oil cooking spray. Flip them when the bottoms start to brown. Since there's no oil in this recipe, don't overcook them or they'll get tough.

VARIATION: Immediately after you've put the batter into the hot skillet, drop in some slices of fresh fruit. Bananas, strawberries, blueberries, and apples are recommended.
  Don't try this batter in your waffle maker. The batter stays moist and makes limp waffles.

Our bodies crave complex carbohydrates for breakfast. That's why grains are so popular in breakfast foods. Breakfast bread hot from the oven puts you in a good mood all day. Most of these recipes are so quick, you'll scarcely have time to scald your mouth on your coffee.

1-2-3-4-5 SPICEBREAD
▾ ▾ ▾ ▾ ▾ ▾ ▾

This is a breakfast, tea, or dessert bread. Its exotic flavor comes from two neglected spices: cardamom and coriander. Both are available at most larger grocery stores. They contribute an almost lemony quality that intensifies the 7-Up.

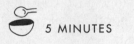 5 MINUTES   55 MINUTES

MAKES 10 SERVINGS.

Preheat oven to **400°F.** In a medium bowl, mix:

> **1 can 7-Up soda**
> **1 teaspoon ground coriander**
> **1 teaspoon ground cardamom**
> **½ cup honey**
> **3 cups Self-Rising Flour** (page 136; or Health-Rising Flour, page 135)

Pour the batter into a loaf pan that's been lightly coated with vegetable oil cooking spray.

Bake for **50 minutes.**

VARIATION: Add ½ cup dates, golden raisins, or figs to the batter.

Hash browns don't have to be soaked in grease. Some tips:

Use cooking spray instead of oil or grease.

Use a grater to shred your potatoes. They'll cook more quickly.

Cook the potatoes for a while before adding onions. Onions burn quickly, so turn frequently with a spatula.

Best of all, use the recipe for fat-free fries on page 18. Cube baked potatoes, dip in egg whites mixed with minced onions, and broil until crisp and brown.

1-2-3-4-5 CITRUS BREAD

A combination of 7-Up and orange juice concentrate makes this dessert bread tangy. It's good sprinkled with a little powdered sugar.

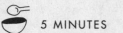 5 MINUTES   55 MINUTES

MAKES 10 SERVINGS.

Preheat oven to **400°F.**

In a medium bowl, mix:

> **1 can 7-Up soda**
> **½ cup orange juice concentrate**
> **3 cups Self-Rising Flour** (page 136; or Health-Rising
>   Flour, page 135)

Pour the batter into a loaf pan that's been lightly coated with vegetable oil cooking spray.

Bake for **50 minutes.**

1-2-3-4-5 Cinnamon Bread

▼▼▼▼▼▼▼

When someone tells you they're dropping by in an hour for coffee, pop a loaf of cinnamon bread in the oven. It gives you time to clean the house, too, before you have to put on the coffee. People are always amazed when you serve hot fresh-baked bread on such short notice.

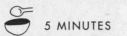 5 MINUTES   55 MINUTES

MAKES 10 SERVINGS.

Preheat oven to **400°F.**

In a medium bowl, mix:

1 can vanilla cream soda
½ cup sorghum molasses (or corn syrup)
3 cups Self-Rising Flour (page 136; or Health-Rising Flour, page 135)
1 tablespoon ground cinnamon

Pour the batter into a loaf pan that's been lightly coated with vegetable oil cooking spray.

Sprinkle with:

¼ cup brown sugar

Bake for **50 minutes.**

VARIATION: Add 1 cup of diced apples, ½ cup dates, or ½ cup golden raisins to the batter. You can also bathe slices of the bread in The Frosting That Moves Like a Sloth (page 41).

ULTRA-CRUNCH GRANOLA

▼▼▼▼▼▼▼

Regular granola and müesli cereals are surprisingly fattening, because they contain nuts and because of the oil used to bind them. Try a cup of this fat-free granola instead. Lighter than typical granola, it's sweet and contains plenty of fruit.

A bowlful with skim milk makes a quick, filling breakfast. And it's an addictive nonfattening snack.

 15 MINUTES   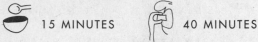 40 MINUTES

MAKES FIFTEEN ½-CUP SERVINGS.

Preheat oven to **250°F.**

In a large bowl, mix:

> **⅓ cup brown sugar**
> **¼ cup honey**
> **1 teaspoon vanilla extract**
> **2 tablespoons nonfat non-instant dry milk**
> (available at health food stores)
> **½ teaspoon salt**
> **2 tablespoons water**

Stir well. Add:

> **2 cups mixed dried fruit** (chopped dates, golden raisins, currants, dried apples, banana chips)

Stir. Add:

> **1 cup Cheerios** or **Oat Flakes**

Stir. Add:

> **4 cups Puffed Rice**

Stir. Spread onto a nonstick cookie sheet.

Bake for **25 minutes,** stirring every 5 minutes.

Remove from oven and let cool.

Your body requires fifteen to twenty-five grams of fat a day to survive. Try to fill your quota with good fat, that is, *unsaturated* fat. There are two varieties: polyunsaturated fat (vegetable and seed oils) and monounsaturated fat (olive oil). These contain no cholesterol.

BAD FAT IS SATURATED FAT: Animal fats (like full-fat dairy products) and tropical oils (coconut and palm kernel). To avoid saturated fat, eat leaner meat and less of it, and low-fat dairy products.

Remember that any fat is bad fat if it's cascading over your waist.

SHAKER BREAD PUDDING WITH OOZING CARAMEL SAUCE

▼ ▼ ▼ ▼ ▼ ▼ ▼

Bread pudding is a Shaker favorite. It's a satisfying breakfast or dessert, and an excellent use of stale bread.

 20 MINUTES   1 HOUR 20 MINUTES

MAKES 10 SERVINGS.

Preheat oven to **350°F.**

In a medium bowl, mix:

4 egg whites
½ cup skim milk
¾ cup sugar
½ cup applesauce (optional)
1 teaspoon vanilla extract
1 tablespoon lemon juice
2 teaspoons ground cinnamon
¼ teaspoon salt

Place **10 slices fat-free bread** (see page 70), crumbled, into a loaf pan that's been lightly coated with vegetable oil cooking spray. Top with liquid mixture.

Bake for **70 minutes.**

While it's baking, prepare the sauce. In a saucepan, mix:

1 cup brown sugar
½ cup Karo syrup
a pinch of salt

Boil 1 minute. Remove from heat and stir in:

4 tablespoons nonfat non-instant dry milk

When the pudding is done, serve smothered in sauce.

Note: For a lighter pudding, omit the applesauce.

LET'S GET INTIMATE WITH VANILLA

FFJFCB: Vanilla, thank you for consenting to this interview.

VANILLA: Don't mention it.

FFJFCB: So give us some background. Where do you come from?

VANILLA: Personally, I come from Madagascar, where the finest vanilla orchids grow.

FFJFCB: I thought you were from Mexico.

VANILLA: Well, some of my family members do come from Mexico. But they're of suspect quality and cheap taste. The standards are much lower in Mexico. If it doesn't say "Madagascar Bourbon" on the label, then it's probably not as classy as I am.

FFJFCB: What about vanilla flavoring?

VANILLA: Plehh!! Cheap imitations!

FFJFCB: Sorry, we didn't mean to hit a nerve.

VANILLA: Do you know where imitation vanilla comes from? It's a discarded by-product of the paper industry!

FFJFCB: So your recommendation to our readers is to buy only real vanilla?

VANILLA: Oh, no. Some folks like fermented wood juice in their cookies. Let them eat cake with pulp refinery backwash in it!

FFJFCB: Prima donna spice.

VANILLA: What was that?

FFJFCB: Nothing. Thank you.

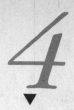

Sweet Treats

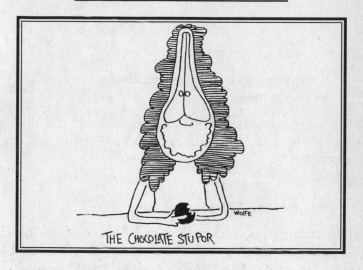

THE CHOCOLATE STUPOR

- ► **RICE KRISPIE TREATS**
- ► **ROCKY ROAD BROWNIES**
- ► **DATE COOKIE BARS**
- ► **GOOD OL' SUGAR COOKIES**
- ► **GUILTLESS HOLIDAY COOKIES**
- ► **CHOCOLATE ICEBREAK COOKIES**
- ► **CREAMY CHOCOLATE FUDGE**
- ► **CHOCOLATE CHUNK COOKIES**

RICE KRISPIE TREATS

▼▼▼▼▼▼▼

Rice Krispie Treats are easy and quick to throw together. You'll find it hard to tell this fat-free version from the original.

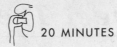 20 MINUTES

MAKES 20 SERVINGS.

In a medium saucepan, place:

4 cups miniature marshmallows
¼ cup buttermilk

Melt over low heat. Once the marshmallows are dissolved, turn the heat up to medium. Boil for **3 minutes,** stirring constantly. Remove from heat.

Add:

5 cups Rice Krispies cereal

Using a large spoon lightly squirted with vegetable oil cooking spray, stir until the cereal is coated. Scoop into a 9 by 13-inch pan that's been lightly coated with vegetable oil cooking spray. Press flat with the spoon. Refrigerate until cool. Cut into 2-inch squares.

VARIATION: Four cups Cocoa Krispies can be used in place of the Rice Krispies.

ROCKY ROAD BROWNIES

▼ ▼ ▼ ▼ ▼ ▼ ▼

This is a deluxe brownie, pretty enough to serve to guests. Its gooey center comes from the marshmallow creme.

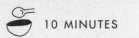 10 MINUTES   30 MINUTES

MAKES 12 BROWNIES.

Preheat oven to **325°F.**

In a medium bowl, combine the following ingredients, one at a time. Beat well after each addition:

4 egg whites
½ cup sugar
1 tablespoon vanilla extract
½ cup cocoa
½ teaspoon baking powder
½ teaspoon salt
½ cup flour

Next, mix in **1 cup marshmallow creme,** just enough so it creates brown and white swirls. Spoon into a 9 by 13-inch pan that's been lightly coated with vegetable oil cooking spray. (For thicker brownies, use a 9 by 9-inch pan.)

Bake for **18 minutes** (20 minutes for a cakey brownie). Cool and serve.

FOOLING FAT

Your body is a fat storage machine. It stockpiles fat to burn in times of need, easily coverting stored fat into energy. By reducing your fat intake, you don't give your body enough dietary fat to store. You also encourage your body to call on stored fat, rather than new, dietary fat, for energy. Repetitive endurance activities, such as bicycling, swimming, running, cross-country skiing, even walking, force your body to burn stored fat.

DATE COOKIE BARS

▼ ▼ ▼ ▼ ▼ ▼ ▼

Date bars are chewy cookie bars that make a fine addition to dessert trays. They keep well in a tin, so it's always nice to have a batch on hand for unexpected guests.

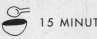 15 MINUTES 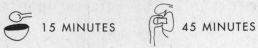 45 MINUTES

MAKES 12 SERVINGS.

Preheat oven to **325°F.**

In a medium bowl, put:

4 egg whites

Beat until foamy. Add the following ingredients one at a time, mixing well after each addition:

½ cup sugar
½ teaspoon vanilla extract
½ teaspoon baking powder
½ teaspoon salt
½ cup flour
2 cups chopped dates

Spoon the batter into a 9 by 13-inch nonstick pan that's been lightly coated with vegetable oil cooking spray.

Bake for **25 to 30 minutes,** until the top starts to brown.

Let cool. Sprinkle top with **powdered sugar.** Cut into 1¼-inch squares.

Store in a tin.

Good Ol' Sugar Cookies

▼▼▼▼▼▼▼

Sugar cookies are good for filling cookie jars. Whenever kids drop by, or you just want a little something sweet, or you need something to fill out lunches, they come in handy.

 20 MINUTES 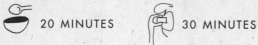 30 MINUTES

MAKES 2 TO 3 DOZEN COOKIES; EIGHT COOKIES CONTAIN LESS THAN ONE-HALF GRAM OF FAT.

Preheat oven to **325°F.**

In a medium bowl, mix the following ingredients one at a time. Blend well after each addition:

2 egg whites
1 cup sugar
1 teaspoon baking powder
a pinch of salt
1 teaspoon vanilla extract
1 cup flour

Drop by teaspoonfuls onto a cookie sheet that's been lightly coated with vegetable oil cooking spray. Sprinkle tops of cookies with **sugar, coarse sugar, turbinado sugar,** or **colored sugar.**

Bake for **9 to 12 minutes.** Cool about 3 minutes before removing from the sheet.

VARIATION: Add 1 teaspoon ground cinnamon.

Guiltless Holiday Cookies

▼▼▼▼▼▼▼

Not only can this basic cookie dough be cut with a cookie cutter, it can also be modified to make numerous kinds of cookies. When the cookies are eaten warm, they're moist and chewy. When cool, they get crispy on the outside and stay chewy inside.

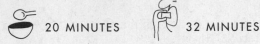 20 MINUTES   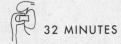 32 MINUTES

MAKES 6 DOZEN COOKIES; ONE DOZEN CONTAINS LESS THAN ONE-HALF GRAM OF FAT.

Preheat oven to **325°F.**

In a medium bowl, mix the following ingredients one at a time until well blended:

> **2 egg whites**
> **1 cup sugar**
> **1 cup honey**
> **1 tablespoon vinegar**
> **1 tablespoon vanilla extract**
> **1 tablespoon baking soda**
> **4 to 5 cups flour**

The dough will be thick (the consistency of cold Play-Doh). Sprinkle ¼ cup flour on a work surface. Dump dough on top and sprinkle with enough flour to keep it from sticking to your rolling pin. Roll flat to ¼-inch thickness. Cut with cookie cutters and place on a nonstick cookie sheet that's been covered with wax paper.

Bake for **12 minutes.** Let cool 5 minutes before removing.

VARIATIONS: For a heartier taste and darker cookie, use raw honey, sorghum, or blackstrap molasses instead of regular honey. The texture of the cookie can be changed by using unbleached flour or a combination of whole wheat pastry flour and unbleached white flour.

COOKIE BARS: Add some chopped dates and golden raisins to the batter. Spread into a sheet cake pan that's been sprayed with vegetable oil cooking spray and dusted with flour. Bake 30 minutes.

GINGER COOKIES: Add 1 tablespoon ground ginger or fresh grated ginger to the dough. The dough holds up well enough to make gingerbread people and gingerbread houses.

CINNAMON COOKIES: Add 1 tablespoon ground cinnamon and ¼ teaspoon ground cloves to the dough.

CHOCOLATE COOKIES: Cut the flour by ½ cup. Add ½ cup cocoa and ½ teaspoon ground cinnamon. (With the addition of cocoa, the fat-free serving size is cut to 4 cookies.)

► QUICK COOKIE FROSTING ◄

This simple recipe for powdered-sugar frosting is also flexible.

Mix:

3 tablespoons hot water
2½ cups powdered sugar

Stir until smooth. Spread onto cookies or squirt through a cake decorating tube.

VANILLA FROSTING: Instead of the water, add 2 tablespoons hot water and 1 tablespoon vanilla extract to the powdered sugar.

ORANGE FROSTING: Instead of water, use 3 tablespoons orange juice concentrate or 3 tablespoons orange liqueur. Try this frosting on ginger, cinnamon, or chocolate cookies.

MINT FROSTING: Instead of the water, use 2 tablespoons plus 2 teaspoons hot water, 1 teaspoon mint extract, and a few drops of green food coloring (or 3 tablespoons crème de menthe). Goes well with chocolate cookies.

LEMON FROSTING: Skip the water; use 3 tablespoons lemon juice and maybe a few drops of yellow food coloring.

COFFEE FROSTING: Instead of water, use 3 tablespoons hot strong coffee. Good on ginger, cinnamon, or chocolate cookies.

CHOCOLATE ICEBREAK COOKIES

▼▼▼▼▼▼▼

These are a chocolate lover's dream. They're elegant enough to serve at a formal tea. They're fun to make, so kids love to help. They're like a brownie in a cookie, only lighter. The name "Icebreak" comes from the powdered sugar coating the cookie gets before baking. As the cookie bakes, it flattens, and the sugar breaks into patches that look like broken ice. These are refrigerator batter cookies, so the dough needs to chill overnight. The advantage to this kind of cookie is that once the dough is chilled, you can bake them fifteen minutes before serving. They're best hot, so it's a good idea to bake as you need. The batter keeps about a week in the refrigerator.

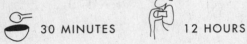 30 MINUTES   12 HOURS

MAKES 3 DOZEN COOKIES; ONE COOKIE CONTAINS LESS THAN ONE-HALF GRAM OF FAT.

In a medium saucepan, mix:

> ³⁄₄ **cup buttermilk**
> ³⁄₄ **cup cocoa**

Heat on medium, stirring constantly until the liquid starts to thicken (about 1 minute). Remove from heat. Pour into a large bowl and add:

> **2¹⁄₂ cups sugar**
> **8 egg whites**
> **2 teaspoons vanilla extract**

Beat until smooth. Stir in:

> **2¹⁄₂ cups flour**
> **2 teaspoons baking powder**
> **¹⁄₂ teaspoon salt**

Chill overnight in the refrigerator.

When you're ready to serve, preheat oven to **350°F.** Drop spoonfuls of the dough into a bowl filled with:

1 cup powdered sugar

Cover each ball completely with sugar. Drop onto a cookie sheet that's been treated with a light coat of vegetable oil cooking spray.

Bake for **10 minutes.**

Remove promptly from the sheet, place on serving plate, and eat while they're hot.

CREAMY CHOCOLATE FUDGE

▼▼▼▼▼▼▼

Some call making fudge a precise art. Some call it an exacting science. Most call it a total pain. The recipe is simple; it's the preparation that's tricky. But if you're a chocolate lover, there's no doubt it's worth the trouble.

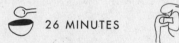 26 MINUTES  1 HOUR

MAKES 8 SERVINGS.

In a large saucepan, mix:

> **2 cups sugar**
> **2 tablespoons corn syrup**
> **¼ cup cocoa**
> **½ cup skim milk**

Set on a burner over **medium-low** heat.

Stir constantly until the sugar is dissolved. (CAUTION: One grain of undissolved sugar can turn the whole batch bad. Scrape the sides of your saucepan with your spoon regularly.)

Once you stop hearing the crunching sound of sugar under your spoon as you stir, and cease to feel the grit, turn the heat up to medium. Stir constantly as you bring it to a boil. The fudge is done when you can pick up with your fingers a ball of the mixture dropped in cold water. Test regularly. When it's passed the test, stop stirring and remove from heat.

Add:

> **1 tablespoon vanilla extract** and let cool (DO NOT stir while cooling. This can make the fudge turn to sugar.)

Beating the fudge at the exact time in the cooling process is vital. If you have a candy thermometer, the exact time is when the fudge cools to 110°F. If you don't have a thermometer, this moment is about 15 to 20 minutes into the cooling process, when the fudge starts to thicken. Another method is to touch the side of the pan. The fudge is done when I can comfortably hold the sides of my Magnalite pan for 10 seconds.

At this point, using a wooden spoon, beat the fudge thoroughly and pour it into a bread pan that's been lightly coated with vegetable oil cooking spray. Continue cooling until firm.

CHOCOLATE CHUNK COOKIES

▼▼▼▼▼▼

Half of every real chocolate chip you eat is fat. Some companies use imitation chocolate flavoring, paraffin, and probably space-age polymers, but most still haven't managed to get the fat content below 40 percent. These cookies use fat-free fudge as a substitute for real chocolate chips.

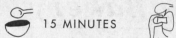 15 MINUTES   30 MINUTES

MAKES 4 DOZEN COOKIES; ONE COOKIE CONTAINS JUST UNDER ONE-HALF GRAM OF FAT.

Preheat oven to **325°F.**

In a large bowl, mix:

> **¼ cup buttermilk**
> **1 cup sugar**

Mix in the following ingredients one at a time, stirring well after each addition:

> **1 cup brown sugar**
> **4 egg whites**
> **1 tablespoon vanilla extract**
> **1½ cups flour**
> **1 teaspoon baking soda**
> **2 teaspoons baking powder**
> **4 cups oats**

Drop by teaspoonfuls onto a nonstick cookie sheet that's been lightly coated with vegetable oil cooking spray.

Cut ½-inch squares of **Creamy Chocolate Fudge** (pages 61–62) and place in a layer on top of the cookies.

Bake for **13 minutes.**

Note: Hershey's Reduced Fat Chips can be used in chocolate chip cookies with wonderful results; however, this raises the fat content to one gram per cookie.

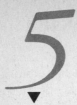

Fresh from the Bakery

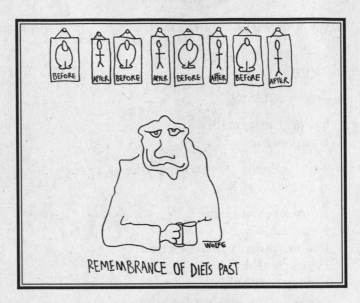

REMEMBRANCE OF DIETS PAST

- ▶ **ULTRALIGHT PASTRY DOUGH**

- ▶ **DOWNY BREADSTICKS**

- ▶ **WINNER DINNER ROLLS**

- ▶ **ANTI-GRAVTIY BISCUITS**

- ▶ **SWEET WHITE BREAD**

- ▶ **GUARANTEED FOUL-MOUTH GARLIC TOAST**

- ▶ QUICK BUTTERMILK BISCUITS

- ▶ UNIVERSAL QUICKBREAD

- ▶ 1-2-3-4-5 BEERBREAD

- ▶ 1-2-3-4-5 CRACKED PEPPER BREAD

- ▶ 1-2-3-4-5 IRISH SODA OAT BREAD

ULTRALIGHT PASTRY DOUGH

▼▼▼▼▼▼

A massive quantity of butter is what makes pastry so fattening. Butter contains eleven grams of fat per tablespoon, so a large butter pastry can take up a whole day's allotment of fat. Fortunately, there's an alternative. This sweet, delicate yeast dough can be used for everything from fat-free cinnamon rolls to fat-free cheese danishes.

No machinery is involved in making this dough; it's just you and the bread. You'll find the mixing, kneading, and rolling by hand therapeutic. It gives you a kinship to your creation, in a Shirley Maclaine kind of way. Don't try this recipe in a bread machine. Not only is it sacrilege, but it doesn't work.

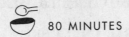 80 MINUTES

In a large bowl, mix:

> **1⅓ tablespoons yeast**
> **1 cup lukewarm skim milk**

Stir gently for about a minute. The yeast will not completely dissolve in milk. That's normal.

Mix in:

> **¼ cup sugar**
> **1½ cups flour** (a soft winter-wheat flour like White Lily is best)
> **2 egg whites**

Stir 100 strokes. Let rise for **30 minutes.**

Mix in:

> **1 teaspoon salt**
> **1⅓ cups flour**

Stir until well mixed. (The dough will start pulling away from the sides of the bowl.) With a little additional flour sprinkled on the dough, knead for 5 minutes.

Let rise for **40 minutes.**

The dough is now ready to be used for: Golden Flatbread (page 30), Wicked Cinnamon Rolls (pages 40–41), Sweet Cheese Puffs (page 42), Downy Breadsticks (below), Winner Dinner Rolls (pages 68–69), Anti-Gravity Biscuits (page 69), or Sweet White Bread (page 70).

DOWNY BREADSTICKS
▼ ▼ ▼ ▼ ▼ ▼ ▼

Soft breadsticks are a wonderful complement to pasta and red sauce. If you want to keep these fat-free, you can't dip them in butter. But there are some options. You can dip them in Scorching Nachos sauce (page 24). Or leave off the garlic and dip them in a chocolate fondue (page 113).

 50 MINUTES   2 HOURS 10 MINUTES

MAKES 12 SERVINGS OF 2 BREADSTICKS EACH.

Make **Ultralight Pastry Dough** (opposite) through the second rise.

Preheat oven to **375°F.**

Grab hunks of dough the size of golf balls. You should have 24 in all. On a floured surface, roll each into a stick about ½ inch across and 6 to 8 inches long. Lay on a cookie sheet that's been lightly coated with vegetable oil cooking spray.

Brush the tops with **egg wash** (1 egg white mixed with 2 tablespoons skim milk). Sprinkle on some **garlic powder,** if you like.

Let rise for **20 minutes.**

Bake for **15 minutes** or until the tops are golden brown.

Serve warm.

WINNER DINNER ROLLS

▼▼▼▼▼▼▼

Elegant, slightly sweet, light and tender. They certainly don't taste fat-free, but they are.

 50 MINUTES   2 HOURS 50 MINUTES

MAKES 12 SERVINGS OF 2 ROLLS EACH.

Make **Ultralight Pastry Dough** (pages 66–67) through the second rise.

FOR ROUND DINNER ROLLS: With floured hands, grab pieces of dough a little larger than a golf ball. Roll into 24 balls. Place about 3 inches apart on nonstick cookie sheets that have been lightly coated with vegetable oil cooking spray. Brush the tops with egg wash (1 egg white mixed with 2 tablespoons skim milk).

FOR CRESCENT ROLLS: Sprinkle flour onto a work surface. Place the dough on top and sprinkle with enough flour to keep it from sticking to your rolling pin. Roll the dough flat until it's about ¼ inch thick. Cut into 24 triangles about 6 inches long and 4 inches wide at the base. Starting at the base end, roll up. Place about 4 inches apart on nonstick cookie sheets that have been lightly coated with vegetable oil cooking spray. Bend ends in to make a crescent shape or further to touch each other. Brush tops with egg wash (1 egg white mixed with 2 tablespoons water).

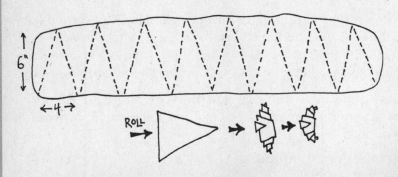

Preheat oven to **375°F.**

Let rolls rise for **20 minutes.**

Bake for **15 minutes** until the tops are golden.

Note: After the rolls are formed and brushed with the egg wash, they can be frozen and baked any time. No need for thawing, just place them on a cookie sheet and bake for 20 minutes or until the tops are light golden.

ANTI-GRAVITY BISCUITS

▼ ▼ ▼ ▼ ▼ ▼ ▼

These biscuits are light and tender—great for Sunday mornings when an epidemic of guests shows up. The three risings give you plenty of time to fix everything else you need for a large breakfast or brunch.

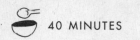 40 MINUTES 2 HOURS 35 MINUTES

MAKES 9 SERVINGS OF 2 BISCUITS EACH.

Make **Ultralight Pastry Dough** (pages 66–67) through the second rise.

Sprinkle flour onto a work surface. Place the dough on top and sprinkle with enough flour to keep it from sticking to your rolling pin.

Roll the dough flat until it's about ½ inch thick. Cut with a biscuit cutter or a drinking glass. Place on a nonstick cookie sheet.

Preheat the oven to **375°F.**

Let rise for **20 minutes.**

Bake for **15 minutes** until the tops are light golden. Don't overbake or the biscuits will get tough and chewy.

Note: After the biscuits are shaped, they can be frozen and baked any time. No need for thawing, just place them on a cookie sheet and bake for 20 minutes or until tops are light golden.

SWEET WHITE BREAD

▼▼▼▼▼▼▼

This is a creamy, light, sweet white bread that's worth the morning it takes to bake it. You can triple the recipe to make three loaves and freeze two for later. The bread is sweet and light enough that it tastes like a pastry. But it's not too sweet to be used for sandwiches, garlic bread, or French toast.

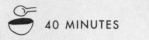 40 MINUTES   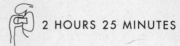 2 HOURS 25 MINUTES

EACH LOAF MAKES SIX 2-SLICE SERVINGS.

Make **Ultralight Pastry Dough** (pages 66–67) through the second rise.

Preheat oven to **350°F.**

Place dough in a nonstick bread pan. Push the dough flat.

Let rise for **20 minutes.**

Brush top of loaf with **egg wash** (1 egg white mixed with 2 tablespoons skim milk).

Bake for **45 minutes.**

GUARANTEED FOUL-MOUTH GARLIC TOAST

▼▼▼▼▼▼▼

Spaghetti with marinara sauce makes a hearty low-fat meal. The pitfall: Eating butter-laden garlic bread along with it.

This fat-free recipe is fancy enough to serve to guests, but even simpler to make than regular garlic bread.

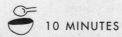 10 MINUTES

MAKES 6 SERVINGS.

Start with:

6 thick slices fat-free white bread (if you can't find any fat-free bread you like in the store, see Sweet White Bread, opposite)

Place on a cookie sheet. Lightly coat the bread with:

vegetable oil cooking spray or fat-free margarine spray

Sprinkle **garlic powder** lightly over bread.

Then sprinkle **Italian seasoning** (oregano, thyme, sage, rosemary, and basil) lightly on top.

Toast under the broiler until the edges start to brown. It can also be toasted in the toaster. (Warning: The toaster method can get messy if you go heavy on the garlic or herbs.)

OPTION: Instead of toasting, wrap the seasoned slices in foil. Put in the oven at 325°F. for 15 minutes.

QUICK BUTTERMILK BISCUITS

▼▼▼▼▼▼▼

The disaster of unexpected breakfast guests is usually a lot worse than the disaster of unexpected dinner guests. For dinner, you can often just set another plate. But for breakfast, you often weren't having any.

It's less than 20 minutes from the time the breakfast guest panic alarm goes off until these biscuits are on the table. They also go well with hearty dinners.

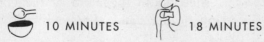 10 MINUTES   18 MINUTES

MAKES 13 FAT-FREE BISCUITS.

Preheat oven to **500°F.**

In a medium bowl, mix:

> **2 cups Self-Rising Flour** (page 136; or Health-Rising
> Flour, page 135)
> **1 cup buttermilk**

The dough will still look moist. Remove from bowl with a spatula and place on a floured surface. Sprinkle more flour on top. Flatten with your hands.

Remember: Biscuits are shy. The more you fuss over them, the less they rise. For the lightest biscuits possible, mix with just a few strokes and don't knead them.

Cut biscuits with a cutter or drinking glass and place on a nonstick cookie sheet. Bake for **8 minutes** (that's not a typo, 8 minutes is correct). As with all fat-free recipes, don't overbake or the biscuits will get tough.

Quickbreads

If making bread is a mystical experience, making quickbread is a sleight-of-hand act. The illusion is that you've spent hours mixing, kneading, and baking a loaf of bread. The magician's secret is that your quickbread took about 3 minutes to make and 50 minutes to bake.

These are probably the simplest bread recipes you'll find. Mix one up, stick it in the oven, make dinner, and your bread will be ready about the same time you're putting the food on the table. If you're really in a rush, the bread can be mixed right in the prepared loaf pan.

If you're concerned about the alum or bleached wheat found in self-rising flours, make them with Health-Rising Flour (page 135).

UNIVERSAL QUICKBREAD

▼▼▼▼▼▼▼

The premise of Universal Quickbread is simple and very flexible.

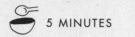 5 MINUTES   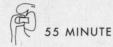 55 MINUTES

MAKES 10 SERVINGS.

Preheat oven to **400°F.**

Mix:

- **1 can of something that fizzes** (club soda, soft drinks, or beer)
- **2 tablespoons of something sweet** (sugar, honey, molasses, syrup, or fruit juice concentrate)
- **3 cups Self-Rising Flour** (page 136; or Health-Rising Flour, page 135)

Put in a loaf pan that has been lightly sprayed with vegetable oil cooking spray and bake for **50 minutes.**

You can eat the bread right out of the oven when it's still crumbly and hot. For nice slices, let it cool 20 minutes. For a flatter bread, bake in a 9 by 5-inch loaf pan. If you want a sandwich loaf, bake it in an 8½ by 4½-inch loaf pan.

Note: You can add fresh fruit to the sweeter bread batters like spicebread (see page 47), citrus bread (see page 48), and cinnamon bread (see page 49). You can also make muffins out of the batter in a muffin tin

---

BURNING OFF THE FAT: THE RIGHT EXERCISE

Recent research shows that certain exercises burn more fat than others.

Jerky, quick exercises like tennis and weight lifting burn a fuel mixture of about one-third fat. Steady, traveling exercises like walking, swimming, race walking, running, bicycling, and cross-country skiing burn a fuel mixture of more than half fat.

Want to lose weight? Take a hike!

1-2-3-4-5 BEERBREAD

▼▼▼▼▼▼▼

Beerbread is a very "yeasty" tasting bread. The beer gives it a traditional bread taste and smell, but there's no yeast in the recipe. Beerbread goes well with soups.

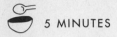 5 MINUTES 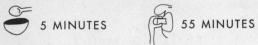 55 MINUTES

MAKES 10 SERVINGS.

Preheat oven to **400°F.**

In a medium bowl, mix:

1 can beer (any kind)
2 tablespoons honey
3 cups Self-Rising Flour (page 136; or Health-Rising Flour, page 135)

Pour batter into a loaf pan that's been lightly coated with vegetable oil cooking spray.

Bake for **50 minutes.**

1-2-3-4-5 CRACKED PEPPER BREAD

▼▼▼▼▼▼▼

Ginger ale and pepper blend to give this bread a biscuity flavor. There's no need to add a sweetener to the batter; the sugar in the ginger ale takes care of that. It's a good bread to toast for sandwiches. It can be baked in a muffin tin for quick biscuits (just cut the baking time to 15 to 20 minutes).

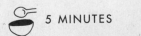 5 MINUTES 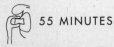 55 MINUTES

MAKES 10 SERVINGS.

Preheat oven to **400°F.**

In a medium bowl, mix:

> **1 can ginger ale** (Vernor's is recommended)
> **2 teaspoons coarse-ground black pepper**
> **3 cups Self-Rising Flour** (page 136; or Health-Rising
> Flour, page 135)

Pour batter into a loaf pan that's been lightly coated with vegetable oil cooking spray.

Bake for **50 minutes.**

1-2-3-4-5 IRISH SODA OAT BREAD

▼▼▼▼▼▼▼

Oats make this bread light, but hearty. Bake a loaf for dinner. The next morning, slice and toast the leftovers. They're tasty with a little jam or honey.

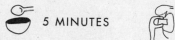 5 MINUTES   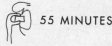 55 MINUTES

MAKES 10 SERVINGS.

Preheat oven to **400°F.**

In a medium bowl, mix:

> **1 can club soda** (must be club soda and not mineral
> water with bubbles blown into it)
> **½ cup molasses** (or corn syrup or sorghum)
> **2½ cups Self-Rising Flour** (page 136; or Health-
> Rising Flour, page 135)
> **½ cup oats** (quick or regular)

Pour batter into an ungreased nonstick loaf pan.

Bake for **50 minutes.**

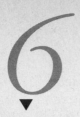

Power Picnicking

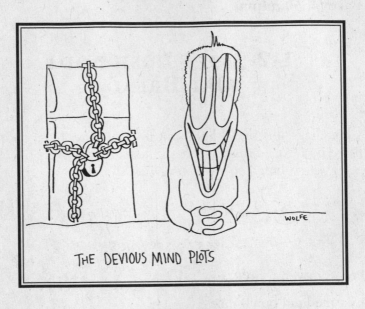

THE DEVIOUS MIND PLOTS

- ▶ **BLUE CHEESE POTATO SALAD**
- ▶ **CREAMY MACARONI SALAD**
- ▶ **DEVIOUS DEVILED EGGS**
- ▶ **BARBECUE BEANS**
- ▶ **CHERRY COKE JELL-O SALAD**
- ▶ **TOTALLY JUNKED AMBROSIA SALAD**

- ► ZESTY COLESLAW
- ► SIZZLING HOT SLAW
- ► SIMPLE INDIA SALAD
- ► GARLIC AND HERB CROUTONS
- ► HONEY DIJON DRESSING
- ► HONEY CATALINA DRESSING
- ► SWEET AND SOUR VINAIGRETTE DRESSING
- ► LUSH ITALIAN DRESSING
- ► HAIL CAESAR DRESSING
- ► REVOLUTIONARY FRENCH DRESSING
- ► COLONIAL HONEY DRESSING
- ► THOUSAND ISLAND DRESSING
- ► FRESH BUTTERMILK RANCH DIP

BLUE CHEESE POTATO SALAD

▼▼▼▼▼▼▼

Potato salad is one of the few salads that everyone eats. Fat-free blue cheese dressing gives this virtuous version a creamy texture and a tangy taste.

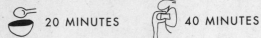 20 MINUTES   40 MINUTES

MAKES 10 SERVINGS.

Peel and cube:

6 medium potatoes

Boil until tender, about **20 minutes.** Drain off the water and set potatoes aside.

In a large bowl, mix:

1 teaspoon dry mustard
⅓ cup fat-free blue cheese dressing
1 teaspoon salt
1 celery stalk (diced)
1 medium onion (diced)
¼ cup of diced red bell pepper
¼ teaspoon black pepper
4 hard-boiled egg whites (chopped)

Mix well. Add the potatoes and stir gently so you don't break them. Serve warm or chilled.

CREAMY MACARONI SALAD

▼▼▼▼▼▼▼

This is the original cold pasta salad. It's good for hot weather, and it contains enough protein to make a satisfying main course.

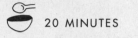 20 MINUTES 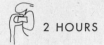 2 HOURS

MAKES 8 SERVINGS.

Boil **2 cups macaroni** until tender. Drain and set aside.

Put the following in a large bowl:

¼ cup nonfat yogurt
¼ cup fat-free mayonnaise
2 tablespoons honey
1 teaspoon salt
¼ cup chopped red bell pepper
¼ cup chopped green onions

Stir in the macaroni and chill before serving.

WHERE FAT'S AT

If a product on your store's shelf doesn't list the fat content, check the list of ingredients for high-fat items. The ingredients at the beginning of the list are the highest in volume: Be most cautious of these.

HIGH-FAT INGREDIENTS: Animal fats, oils, tallow, butter, lard, shortening, margarine, nut butters, nuts, red meat, bacon, mayonnaise, egg yolks, and avocados.

DEVIOUS DEVILED EGGS

▼▼▼▼▼▼

The devious part of these eggs is that they contain no egg yolks. Mustard helps duplicate the missing yolk taste.

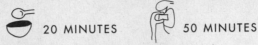 20 MINUTES   50 MINUTES

MAKES 12 DEVILED EGGS; 4 CONTAIN LESS THAN ONE-HALF GRAM OF FAT.

Boil:

6 eggs for about **5 minutes.** Let cool 10 minutes.

In a food processor, place:

1 cup fresh mushroom
3 tablespoons minced onion
1 tablespoon pickle relish
1 garlic clove
¼ teaspoon salt
¼ teaspoon black pepper
3 teaspoons Dijon or yellow mustard
1 teaspoon fat-free mayonnaise

Process until smooth. Slice the hard-boiled eggs in half, lengthwise. Remove the yolks and send them to your in-laws. Fill the cavities with the deviled filling. Chill before serving.

BARBECUE BEANS

▼▼▼▼▼▼▼

Most picnic foods are white, yellow, or green. A few, such as steak and burgers, are nearly black. Baked beans add some much-needed medium tones to the spread. And these taste pretty good, too.

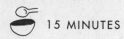 15 MINUTES 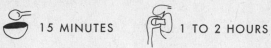 1 TO 2 HOURS

MAKES 9 SERVINGS.

Preheat oven to **350°F.**

In a glass baking dish, mix:

3 15-ounce cans navy beans
1 cup barbecue sauce
3 tablespoons cider vinegar
1 teaspoon dry mustard
1 large onion (chopped)
½ teaspoon Liquid Smoke (optional)

Bake for **1½ hours.** Or microwave on **high** for **30 minutes.** Serve hot or cold.

Tip: Try with some imitation bacon bits on top!

CHERRY COKE JELL-O SALAD

▼▼▼▼▼▼

For those who like a salad loaded with caffeine, this one's for you.

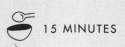 15 MINUTES 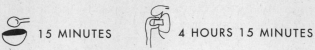 4 HOURS 15 MINUTES

MAKES 10 SERVINGS.

In a large saucepan, pour:

**1 6-ounce package cherry Jell-O
the juice from 1 14.5-ounce can red cherries**
(water-packed)

Mix well. Bring to a boil. Remove from heat and, using an electric mixer, blend in the following ingredients, one at a time, mixing after each:

**1 8-ounce package fat-free cream cheese
20 ounces Coca-Cola** (2½ cups)

Add **the canned cherries.** Mix with a spoon.

Chill for **4 hours.** Serve with Cool Whip Lite, if desired.

TOTALLY JUNKED
AMBROSIA SALAD

▼▼▼▼▼▼▼

What makes this fruit salad so great is the sweet syrup that drowns the fruit. If the fresh fruit you use is off-season, the syrup makes up for its lack of sweetness. Even people who don't like fruit will usually eat this.

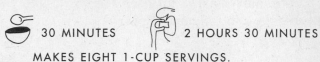 30 MINUTES   2 HOURS 30 MINUTES

MAKES EIGHT 1-CUP SERVINGS.

To make the syrup:

In a medium saucepan, place:

> **2 tablespoons arrowroot powder** (or cornstarch)
> **2 tablespoons water**

Mix until smooth. Add:

> **juice from 2 15-ounce cans fruit** (your choice)
> **water to make 2 cups**
> **¼ cup sugar** (Unless the fruit was packed in heavy syrup. If it was, skip the sugar.)

Boil until clear.

Stir in **1 cup marshmallows.**

While the syrup is cooling, put:

> **the canned fruit** in a serving bowl

Cut up:

> **4 cups fresh fruit** (go for at least six different fruits: strawberries, kiwis, apples, grapes, peaches, pears, melon, tangerines, oranges, blueberries, cherries, or pineapple)

Pour cooled syrup over the mixed fruit. Chill for a few hours before serving.

Note: If you live in a bomb shelter and have no access to fresh fruit, 4 additional 15-ounce drained cans of fruit may be used in place of the fresh fruit.

ZESTY COLESLAW

▼ ▼ ▼ ▼ ▼ ▼ ▼

Most people think of coleslaw as a "healthy" food. Not so. Coleslaw dressings can be as high as 90 percent fat. This recipe is a spicy blend similar to what you find at urban barbecue joints. If you want a milder slaw, drop the horseradish. For a slightly creamier dressing, substitute a quarter cup of fat-free mayonnaise for the yogurt, drop the vinegar, and double the cabbage and the carrots.

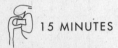 15 MINUTES

MAKES SIX ½-CUP SERVINGS.

In a medium bowl, mix the following:

½ cup plain nonfat yogurt
1 tablespoon vinegar
1 teaspoon horseradish
¼ teaspoon celery seed
2 tablespoons honey
a pinch of salt
½ teaspoon Dijon mustard

Stir well. Pour over:

3 cups shredded cabbage
½ cup shredded carrots

Keep chilled until ready for serving.

Sizzling Hot Slaw

▼ ▼ ▼ ▼ ▼ ▼ ▼

Hot slaw gives you a salad variation for those times of year when cabbage is cheap. Its sweet tangy taste is there, but the bacon grease is gone.

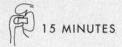 15 MINUTES

MAKES FOUR ½-CUP SERVINGS.

In a large bowl, place:

2 cups finely shredded cabbage
2 tablespoons finely chopped onion
2 tablespoons chopped red bell pepper

Lightly **salt** and **pepper.** Set aside.

In a small saucepan, mix:

1 teaspoon imitation bacon bits
2 tablespoons cider vinegar
2 tablespoons honey

Heat until boiling. Pour on slaw. Toss and serve immediately. If the cabbage is not wilted enough for your taste, microwave for 1 to 2 minutes.

SIMPLE INDIA SALAD

▼ ▼ ▼ ▼ ▼ ▼ ▼

This is a unique salad made from a most common ingredient: iceberg lettuce. Natives of the Indian subcontinent have found a way to flavor iceberg lettuce so there's no need for dressing.

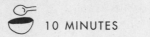 10 MINUTES 1 HOUR

MAKES 4 SERVINGS.

Slice, dice, chop, or rip:

½ head iceberg lettuce

In a large bowl, mix:

3 cups cold water
3 tablespoons lemon juice
2 teaspoons salt

Submerge the lettuce in the bowl. Refrigerate for **30 minutes.** Drain the water. Refrigerate for **20 minutes.** Serve.

READING THE LABEL

What It Says	What It Means
"Fat-Free"	Contains less than one-half gram of fat per serving.
"Low-Fat"	Three grams of fat or less in a fifty-gram serving.
"Lower in Saturated Fat"	Higher in other fats.
"83% Fat-Free"	17% pure fat.
"Saturated Fat/ Unsaturated Fat"	By splitting the fat content, it looks like less.

GARLIC AND HERB CROUTONS

▼▼▼▼▼▼

The croutons you get at the grocery store and in restaurants usually have a lot of oil added to them to make the herbs stick. This recipe uses fat-free bread and vegetable oil cooking spray, which cuts the fat content way down.

 10 MINUTES   30 MINUTES

MAKES TEN ¼-CUP SERVINGS.

Preheat oven to **250°F.**

Cube **6 slices fat-free bread** (see page 70). Place cubes into a large bowl.

On top, sprinkle:

½ teaspoon garlic powder
1 tablespoon Italian herbs (oregano, thyme, sage, rosemary, and basil)

GENTLY toss, with a large spoon. Spray with a two-second burst of vegetable oil cooking spray. Toss. Spray again. Place the cubes on a cookie sheet.

Bake for **20 minutes,** turning frequently, until the cubes are dry. Store in a sealed container.

Any bread may be used, such as whole wheat or rye, but note that this could raise the fat content.

Clothing Your Salads (Dressings)

Don't be fooled: Salads are NOT usually low in fat. True, the salad stuff itself is usually fat-free; it's the dressing that destroys your diet. Commercial dressings contain up to ten grams of fat per tablespoon. And a tablespoon doesn't go very far over a large salad. It's possible that a chef salad with cheese, meat, and an ample amount of dressing can contain more than fifty grams of fat!

You're far better off if you bring your own dressing when attempting a healthy lunch at the salad bar. The dressings that follow skip the oil, but they have the same consistency as an oil-based dressing. Many commercial fat-free dressings are bland and sour. You'll find these from slightly sweet to sweet, and very robust.

HONEY DIJON DRESSING
▼▼▼▼▼▼▼

This tangy dressing can bring even a lowly hunk of iceberg lettuce to life. It's also a great dip for veggies and toasted bagels. Pour some over a baked potato.

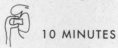 10 MINUTES

MAKES ABOUT EIGHT 2-TABLESPOON SERVINGS.

In a small bowl, mix the following ingredients one at a time. Stir well after each addition:

¼ cup Dijon mustard
2 tablespoons nonfat non-instant dry milk
    (available at health food stores)

THE FAT-FREE JUNK FOOD COOKBOOK

½ teaspoon dry mustard
1 teaspoon onion powder
5 tablespoons honey
¼ cup wine vinegar

Chill before serving.

Note: The dry milk can be omitted. It thickens the dressing and gives it a lighter, more substantial feel.

HONEY CATALINA DRESSING

▼ ▼ ▼ ▼ ▼ ▼ ▼

This red dressing has *punch*. It's sweet, tangy, and hearty. It's so flavorful, you only need to use a little bit. *Toss well.* Use it to baste chicken and pork before grilling. It's also good for giving a kick to sandwiches.

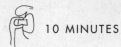 10 MINUTES

MAKES ABOUT SEVEN ¼-CUP SERVINGS.

In a medium bowl, mix:

1 cup ketchup
½ cup honey
2 tablespoons grated onion
1 teaspoon garlic powder
¼ cup vinegar

Keep refrigerated.

Sweet and Sour Vinaigrette Dressing

▼▼▼▼▼▼

Vinaigrette or Italian dressing is usually very high in fat. And if you've tried the fat-free Italian dressings available at the grocery, you've probably been disappointed. They're usually sour, and the flavor of the spices and herbs tends to get lost in your lettuce.

This vinaigrette is fresh, lively, and a bit sweet. It's thin, so if you want a little more body, mix in the Arrowroot Jelly.

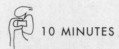 10 MINUTES

MAKES ABOUT EIGHT 1½-TABLESPOON SERVINGS (4 TABLE-SPOONS CONTAIN LESS THAN ONE-HALF GRAM OF FAT).

In a medium bowl, mix:

> **1 cup wine vinegar**
> **1 tablespoon Italian seasoning** (oregano, thyme, sage, rosemary, and basil)
> **2 teaspoons onion powder**
> **2 teaspoons garlic powder**
> **¼ cup honey**
> **2 tablespoons Arrowroot Jelly** (optional; see pages 137–38)

Stir until well blended. Storing this dressing at room temperature brings out the flavor of the herbs.

Lush Italian Dressing

▼▼▼▼▼▼

Fat-free mayonnaise may not have won a lot of people over with its taste, but it works well in salad dressings. This is a nice, light, creamy Italian.

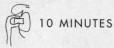 10 MINUTES

MAKES ABOUT SIXTEEN 2-TABLESPOON SERVINGS.

In a medium bowl, mix:

³/₄ cup fat-free mayonnaise
³/₄ cup red wine vinegar
¹/₃ cup water
1 tablespoon Italian seasoning (oregano, thyme, sage, rosemary, and basil)
1¹/₂ teaspoons garlic powder
¹/₃ cup sugar

Using a wire whisk, whip until smooth. Store in the fridge.

HAIL CAESAR DRESSING

▼▼▼▼▼▼

This dressing tastes like an original rich, cheesy caesar dressing. Use on romaine lettuce with some fat-free Parmesan and fat-free Garlic and Herb Croutons (page 87). And you, Brutus, would you like seconds?

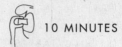 10 MINUTES

MAKES ABOUT NINE 2-TABLESPOON SERVINGS.

In a medium bowl, mix:

½ cup fat-free mayonnaise
½ cup water
2 tablespoons red wine vinegar
1 teaspoon garlic powder
¼ teaspoon Worcestershire sauce
¼ teaspoon black pepper
½ teaspoon salt

Whip with a wire whisk until creamy. Try saying the last sentence six times real fast. Then refrigerate the dressing.

Tip: Adding some fat-free Parmesan cheese gives the dressing a little more bite.

Revolutionary French Dressing

▼ ▼ ▼ ▼ ▼ ▼ ▼

This is a vicious red French dressing. If it's not passionate enough for you, use barbecue sauce instead of ketchup.

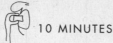 10 MINUTES

MAKES ABOUT TWELVE 2-TABLESPOON SERVINGS.

In a medium bowl, mix:

1 cup ketchup
1 tablespoon dry mustard
¼ cup sugar
½ cup red wine vinegar
1 teaspoon salt
1 teaspoon garlic powder
1 tablespoon Worcestershire sauce

Store in the fridge.

FAT-FREE FOODS YOU MIGHT THINK AREN'T

Marshmallows	Jam	Pickle relish
Marshmallow creme	Preserves	Fruit juice
Hard candy	Ketchup	Soft drinks
Gelatin	Mustard	Beer
Jelly		

These food are all fat-free. But other foods commonly associated with them DO contain a lot of fat.

Marshmallows are associated with s'mores. S'mores are high in fat because of the chocolate. Marshmallow creme is associated with fluffernutter sandwiches. The peanut butter on the sandwich is high in fat. Jelly, jam, and preserves are associated with toast and butter. The butter is high in fat. Ketchup, mustard, and pickle relish are associated with burgers, hot dogs, and fries: All are high in fat. Soft drinks are associated with fried snacks. High in fat. Beer is associated with nuts and nachos. Both are fattening.

Get to know the fat content of what you eat and put the blame where it's due.

COLONIAL HONEY DRESSING

▼▼▼▼▼▼▼

The paprika in this dressing gives it an unexpectedly unexpected taste. It complements light salads made of Bibb, Boston, and the wimpier lettuces. It also goes well on shredded red cabbage and carrots for a radical coleslaw.

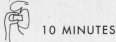 10 MINUTES

MAKES ABOUT EIGHT 2-TABLESPOON SERVINGS.

In a medium bowl, mix:

½ cup red wine vinegar
½ cup honey
1 teaspoon dry mustard
½ teaspoon paprika
1 teaspoon celery seed
½ teaspoon salt
¼ teaspoon onion powder
2 tablespoons Arrowroot Jelly (optional; see pages 136–37)

This dressing doesn't need to be refrigerated. Storing it at room temperature brings out the flavor of the herbs.

Thousand Island Dressing

▼▼▼▼▼▼

The island this dressing comes from is a posh one indeed. The white wine and fresh garlic give an elegant twist to a common dressing. It's one of the thickest Thousand Island dressings you'll find.

Make sure to use some expensive lettuce or artichoke hearts in the salad so the dressing doesn't turn its nose up at the greenery.

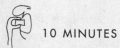 10 MINUTES

MAKES ABOUT TWENTY-TWO 1-TABLESPOON SERVINGS.

In a medium bowl, mix:

1 cup fat-free mayonnaise
2 tablespoons white wine (a sweet German white, such as a Spätlese, is best)
¼ teaspoon paprika
2 finely minced garlic cloves
2 tablespoons ketchup
1 teaspoon fat-free Parmesan cheese

This should be refrigerated.

Fresh Buttermilk Ranch Dip

▼▼▼▼▼▼▼

The fresh buttermilk gives this dressing a "just-made" taste. It keeps about two weeks in the fridge.

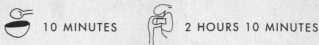 10 MINUTES   2 HOURS 10 MINUTES

PREPARED WITH THE FAT-FREE MAYO, 2 TABLESPOONS ARE
FAT-FREE; WITHOUT: 4 TABLESPOONS ARE FAT-FREE.

In a small bowl, mix the following with a wire whisk:

½ cup buttermilk

2 tablespoons fat-free mayonnaise (optional, for extra thickness and creaminess)

3 tablespoons nonfat non-instant dry milk (available at health food stores)

¼ teaspoon garlic powder

½ teaspoon Italian seasoning (oregano, thyme, sage, rosemary, and basil)

Chill for a few hours to thicken before serving.

Serving Suggestions

◆ Use as a dip for veggies or pretzels.

◆ Use as a marinade and glaze for grilled chicken.

◆ Spread on toasted bagels.

◆ Slather on baked potatoes stuffed with broccoli.

◆ Drizzle over sliced fresh cucumbers for a crunchy salad.

◆ Use like a béarnaise sauce over cooked green vegetables.

THE SHOCKING TRUTH ABOUT BUTTERMILK

The name "buttermilk" is very misleading. Cultured buttermilk is usually only 1 percent butterfat, so it only has two grams of fat per cup. Whole milk has eight grams of fat per cup.

Some types of buttermilk have butterflakes added. Check the label. Only buy buttermilk with three grams of fat per cup or less.

7

Yes, You Can Have Dessert

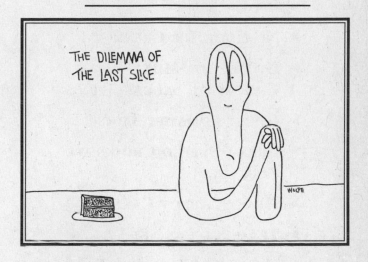

THE DILEMMA OF THE LAST SLICE

WOLFE

- ▶ **CRUNCH COBBLER**

- ▶ **DEATH BY CHOCOLATE AND THEN GONE TO HEAVEN PUDDING**

- ▶ **(THE OBLIGATORY ELVIS RECIPE) 'NANA PUDDIN' FIT FOR THE KING**

- ▶ **RAJAH RICE PUDDING**

- ▶ **DESSERT PIZZA SAUCE**

- ► **Dessert Pizza Blanca Sauce**

- ► **Big Orange Sherbet**

- ► **Intoxicating Sherbet**

- ► **Ice Cream**

- ► **No-Cook Ice Cream**

- ► **Hot Fudgy Milk Chocolate Sauce**

- ► **Gooey Caramel Sauce**

- ► **Cream-Puffed Chocolate Cupcakes**

- ► **Heavy Carrot Cake**

- ► **Texas Sheet Cake**

- ► **Mrs. Lottie's Angel Food Cake**

- ► **Moist Jam Cake**

- ▶ CHOCOLATE THERAPY CAKE

- ▶ GOOEY COCOA CAKE

- ▶ GOOEY SPICE CAKE

- ▶ GOOEY LEMON CAKE

- ▶ WHITE MIRACLE CAKE

- ▶ CHOCOLATE MIRACLE CAKE

- ▶ BUTTERCREAM FROSTING

- ▶ SEVEN-MINUTE FROSTING

- ▶ SWEET YOGURT FROSTING

- ▶ CHOCOLATE BUTTERCREAM FROSTING

- ▶ CREAMY CARAMEL FROSTING

- ▶ RICH BROWNIE FROSTING

- ▶ BANANA EGGNOG

- ▶ HOT SPICED CIDER

CRUNCH COBBLER

▼▼▼▼▼▼▼

Hot apple cobbler baking in the oven. Catch a whiff of warm cinnamon and apples and the whole meal seems more appetizing. So if you have a meal that's not going well in the cooking process, throw an apple cobbler in the oven to salvage it. Peach cobbler can be made with fresh or canned peaches. Cherry-berry cobbler is a refreshing variation if you come into an overabundance of fresh strawberries.

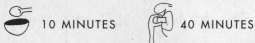 10 MINUTES   40 MINUTES

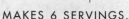

MAKES 6 SERVINGS.

Preheat oven to **350°F.**

Lightly coat a 9 by 9-inch glass baking dish with vegetable oil cooking spray. Cover the bottom of the dish with:

> **2 to 3 cups sliced apples or peaches** or **2 cups fresh strawberries and 1 can cherry pie filling**

In a medium bowl, mix:

> **1 cup flour**
> **1 cup sugar**
> **1 teaspoon baking powder**
> **a pinch of salt**
> **2 egg whites**
> **½ teaspoon ground cinnamon**
> **¼ teaspoon nutmeg**

Spread batter over the fruit until it's covered.

Bake for **30 minutes.**

Note: If making apple cobbler, you might want to up the cinnamon to 1 teaspoon.

Death by Chocolate and Then Gone to Heaven Pudding

▼▼▼▼▼▼▼

Chocolate pudding need not be a fattening dessert. Each serving of this pudding contains less than one-half gram of fat.

You can top it with meringue (see pages 102–103) for an old-fashioned baked pudding.

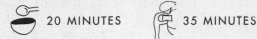 20 MINUTES   35 MINUTES

MAKES 5 SERVINGS.

In a medium saucepan, mix:

1 cup sugar
4 tablespoons cornstarch
¼ teaspoon salt
3 tablespoons cocoa
2 cups skim milk

Stir over medium heat until the pudding starts to thicken. Pour into a medium-size bowl. Chill at least 15 minutes before serving.

VARIATION: To make with meringue topping, pour thickened pudding into an ovenproof dish. Preheat oven to 350° F. Spread meringue over surface of the pudding, mounding in the middle and making sure the meringue extends to the rim of the dish. Bake for 20 minutes, until the meringue is set and lightly browned.

(THE OBLIGATORY ELVIS RECIPE) 'NANA PUDDIN' FIT FOR THE KING

▼ ▼ ▼ ▼ ▼ ▼ ▼

Banana pudding is the perfect dessert to make when you find yourself with a full bunch of overly ripe bananas. When bananas start to get brown spots, they're at their sweetest.

If you like graham crackers or vanilla wafers on the bottom of your banana pudding, line the bottom of the serving dish with six to twelve Guiltless Holiday Cookies (pages 58–59).

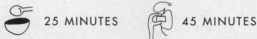 25 MINUTES   45 MINUTES

MAKES 5 SERVINGS (ANY ADDED COOKIES WILL INCREASE THE AMOUNT OF FAT).

Preheat oven to **350°F.**

In a large saucepan, mix:

> **2 cups skim milk**
> **⅔ cup sugar**
> **¼ cup cornstarch**
> **¼ teaspoon salt**

Cook over medium heat until thick. Add:

> **1 teaspoon vanilla extract**

Stir. Slice **3 bananas** into the serving dish. Spoon the pudding on top.

Top with meringue. Using an electric beater, whip:

> **2 egg whites**

Add:

¼ cup sugar
½ teaspoon cream of tartar

Whip until the egg whites form stiff peaks. Top your pudding and brown in the oven for **20 minutes.**

MAKING PIES LOOK SPECIAL WITH MERINGUE

Meringue elevates pies, puddings, and other desserts above the average. Lemon meringue and pumpkin are, like many pies, low-fat by nature, with only their crusts being a problem.
Some tips on meringue:

The stiffer you whip meringue, the better it will keep its shape in the oven. You can make designs in really stiff meringue. You can even write messages in it for pies going to relatives in prison. (Most guards eat cakes to make sure there's not a file in them.)

Add food coloring to meringue for special events. Green for St. Pat's Day. Red, white, and blue for the Fourth of July. Team colors for sports celebrations.

Using egg whites that have warmed to room temperature can get more air in your meringue and make it rise higher.

Meringue's biggest drawback is that it "weeps" or gets condensation on top. To avoid sad-meringue syndrome, turn off the oven when done baking and let the pie cool inside. Note that this will make the top of the meringue a little crusty.

RAJAH RICE PUDDING

▼ ▼ ▼ ▼ ▼ ▼ ▼

Here's something a little exotic and different. It's difficult to describe the taste of cardamom, but if you like cinnamon, you'll probably like it. You'll just have to try it and see. This is one of those dishes that you either love or hate. So if you have a less adventurous palate, you might skip this recipe.

This pudding is good for dessert or breakfast.

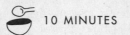 10 MINUTES   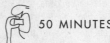 50 MINUTES

MAKES 4 SERVINGS.

In a medium saucepan, mix:

½ cup basmati rice (Texmati brand is good)
2 cups skim milk
⅓ cup honey
¼ teaspoon salt
¼ cup golden raisins
¼ teaspoon ground cardamom

Cover with a lid. Cook over medium-low heat for **40 to 50 minutes.** Stir regularly. After 30 minutes, if there's still a lot of liquid, remove the lid for the rest of the cooking.

Spoon into dishes and cool somewhat before eating.

WHERE DO THEY FIND THESE PEOPLE WHO MAKE THESE DIET CLAIMS?

THE ULTRA-GAUNT FAST DIET: "I lost 312 pounds the first week and I only weighed 205 to start with."

THE HOLLYWOOD HILLS DIET: "I took the pills, I ate all the chocolate I wanted, and now look: I'm a top fashion model."

THE AMAZING FAIRY-TALE DIET: "I ate the yummy magic beans. Not only did I have enough energy to climb the beanstalk, but being chased by that giant is a great exercise program."

Dessert pizza goes over well as a close to dinner, at parties, and for breakfast. It's also a clever way to get people who hate fruit to eat it.

Start with an unbaked K-K-Krispy Pizza Crust (pages 29–30). Preheat oven to **500°F.**

It's best to put the fruit on first, so try any of these fat-free toppings: kiwis, bananas, mangoes, oranges, papayas, pears, pineapples, strawberries, cherries, plums, tangerines, nectarines, dates, figs, apricots, golden raisins, apple butter, or marshmallows.

For an apple, peach, cooked pumpkin, or cooked yam pizza, add 1 teaspoon cinnamon and ¼ teaspoon grated nutmeg to the sauce.

Then pour on one of the sauces below. Bake for 10 minutes. Serve hot.

DESSERT PIZZA SAUCE

▼ ▼ ▼ ▼ ▼ ▼ ▼

This tart, sweet pizza sauce goes particularly well with strawberries, apples, peaches, or bananas.

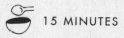 15 MINUTES

MAKES 1 FAT-FREE CUP.

In a medium saucepan, mix:

1 tablespoon arrowroot powder (or cornstarch or flour)

1 cup fruit juice (apple, pineapple, orange, apricot nectar, etc.)

2 tablespoons sugar

Cook over medium heat, stirring constantly, until thick.

DESSERT PIZZA BLANCA SAUCE

▼▼▼▼▼▼▼

This creamy white sauce complements just about any fruit.

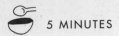 5 MINUTES

MAKES 1 CUP; EACH ¼ CUP CONTAINS LESS THAN
ONE-HALF GRAM OF FAT.

In a small bowl, mix:

> **1 cup fat-free ricotta cheese**
> **¼ cup sugar**
> **a pinch of salt**

VARIATION: Add ¼ teaspoon almond extract to the sauce while mixing. The nutty flavor goes well with apples and peaches.

Blender Iced Desserts

It used to be you had to own an ice cream freezer to make iced desserts. Not anymore. These fat-free frozen desserts can be made and frozen right in your blender. The process is much less involved than making ice cream with an ice cream maker, but it requires that you blend for thirty seconds every hour for about six hours.

Why Ice Cream Is Ice Cream and Not a Lump of Ice

Ice cream needs to be churned to add air and to keep the ice crystals small as they form.

Most of the recipes that follow call for Arrowroot Jelly. It's optional in the sherbets and ice milks, but it's a necessity in the intoxicating sherbets. Since alcohol doesn't freeze well, the jelly is what holds the intoxicating sherbets together. The jelly also adds a creamy texture.

When making these iced desserts in the blender, it's important that you take them out of the freezer and blend them every hour. If you miss an hour, especially the third and fourth hours, you may wind up with an inedible hunk of ice or even a broken blender. It's best to reset your egg timer or an alarm after each blending.

These recipes yield a normal hard-serve iced dessert. For soft-serve: starting at hour three, blend every half-hour for thirty seconds until done. This keeps the ice crystals even smaller.

These recipes can also be made in a regular ice cream freezer. You can double them if your freezer has the capacity.

They can be made without a blender, too. Substitute a freezer-safe container for the blender jar. When the recipe says blend, stir well.

BIG ORANGE SHERBET

▼▼▼▼▼▼▼

 15 MINUTES   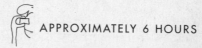 APPROXIMATELY 6 HOURS

MAKES FIVE ½-CUP SERVINGS.

In a blender, mix:

> **6 tablespoons Arrowroot Jelly** (see pages 137–38)
> **12 ounces thawed orange juice concentrate**

When blended, add:

> **2 cups water**

Blend until smooth. Place the glass container of the blender in the freezer, preferably on the bottom shelf where it's colder. Set it in carefully. Make sure it's standing upright and won't fall when you open and close the door.

Remove once an hour for 6 hours. Scrape the sides of the container with a spatula and blend for about 30 seconds. Place back in freezer.

When the mixture is so thick that the blender won't blend it, it's done.

After 6 hours (or 7 if your freezer is warmer), scoop the sherbet into bowls or into a freezer storage container.

Tip: Try topping Orange Sherbet with chocolate sauce (see page 113). Orange and chocolate are a surprisingly complementary flavor combination.

LEMON LIFT SHERBET: Substitute 12 ounces thawed lemonade concentrate for the orange juice concentrate.

FULL-PUCKER LIME SHERBET: Substitute 12 ounces thawed limeade concentrate for the orange juice concentrate. Lime sherbet goes well with lemon cake (see page 123).

INTOXICATING SHERBET
▼▼▼▼▼▼▼

Intoxicating sherbets combine after-dinner drinks with dessert. At roughly thirty proof, they pack a wallop in each scoop. So please: eat responsibly.

The master recipe uses Amaretto, a popular liqueur. The almondy flavor of Amaretto makes it a wonderful addition to chocolate desserts, especially cakes (see pages 120, 121, 126–27). Add a little chocolate syrup on top. Try the variations to find your favorite—or make up your own.

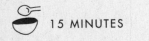 15 MINUTES   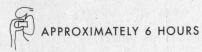 APPROXIMATELY 6 HOURS

MAKES 4 SERVINGS.

In a blender, place:

    2 cups Arrowroot Jelly (see pages 137–38)
    ⅔ cup Amaretto

½ cup sugar
1 teaspoon almond extract or flavoring (not oil-
based)

Blend at high speed for 30 seconds. Put glass blender jar with lid in the freezer, preferably on the bottom shelf, for 3 hours.

Remove, scrape the sides of the jar, and blend at the slowest speed for 30 seconds. Put blender back in the freezer for 2 more hours.

Remove, and scrape sides. Blend on slowest speed for 30 seconds. Put jar back in the freezer for 1 hour.

Scoop into a freezer storage container or serving dishes.

Note: Since alcohol doesn't freeze well, make sure you keep the sherbet stored in the freezer until the moment before you're going to serve it. Serve in chilled bowls. It melts *quickly.*

MOCHA KAHLÚA SHERBET: Substitute ⅔ cup Kahlúa (or other coffee liqueur) and 2 tablespoons instant coffee granules for the Amaretto and almond extract. Mocha Kahlúa Sherbet complements any chocolate dessert.

LEMON JACK SHERBET: Substitute ⅔ cup Yukon Jack and 2 tablespoons lemon juice for the Amaretto and almond extract.

SPICED RUM SHERBET: Substitute ⅔ cup dark rum, 1 cup brown sugar, ¼ teaspoon grated nutmeg, ¼ teaspoon ground cinnamon, and ¼ teaspoon ground cloves for the Amaretto, sugar, and almond extract.

ICE CREAM

▼▼▼▼▼▼

Ice "milk" is such a derogatory term for this ice cream substitute. Even though there's no cream in the recipe, let's lie, since it tastes like there is. This recipe starts out as a thin, cooked pudding. The cooking process makes it look whiter and more appetizing than the pale gray of some fat-free ice cream substitutes and frozen yogurts in your grocer's freezer.

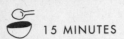 15 MINUTES   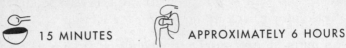 APPROXIMATELY 6 HOURS

MAKES SIX ½-CUP SERVINGS.

In a medium saucepan, combine the following ingredients:

3 egg whites
6 tablespoons arrowroot powder (or cornstarch)
⅓ cup sugar
1 tablespoon vanilla extract
2¼ cups skim milk
¼ teaspoon salt

Stir well over medium-low heat for about 10 to 12 minutes until the mixture starts to thicken. Pour into a blender.

Add:

6 tablespoons nonfat non-instant dry milk
    (available at health food stores)

Blend at slow speed until the dry milk is dissolved.

Place the blender jar in the freezer, preferably on the bottom shelf. Let sit 1 hour. Remove. Scrape the sides of the blender with a rubber spatula. Blend at a slow speed until smooth.

Repeat the scraping and blending each hour for a total of 6 hours.

When the mixture is so thick that the blender won't blend it, it's done.

Spoon the ice milk into a freezer storage container or serving dishes. Keep frozen until ready to serve.

Serving Suggestions

♦ Smother in Hot Fudgy Milk Chocolate Sauce (page 113).

♦ Use thin chocolate Guiltless Holiday Cookies (pages 58–59) to make ice cream sandwiches.

♦ Mix with fruit and skim milk to make a shake or malt.

♦ Slice a banana and top with Hot Fudgy Milk Chocolate Sauce and a cherry for a sinless banana split.

CHOCOLATE ICE CREAM: Add ¼ cup cocoa at the start. At the fifth hour, you can spoon mixture into popsicle molds for fudgesicles. Or keep going for regular chocolate ice cream.

ROCKY ROAD ICE CREAM: Make chocolate ice cream. At the start of the fifth hour, spoon into a freezer container. Mix in miniature marshmallows. Freeze for another hour before eating.

FRENCH VANILLA ICE CREAM: Instead of egg whites, use Egg Beaters equivalent to 3 eggs.

LEMON CHIFFON ICE CREAM: Instead of egg whites, use Egg Beaters equivalent to 3 eggs and add 1 teaspoon lemon extract.

MOCHA ICE CREAM: At the start add 4 tablespoons instant coffee granules.

CHOCOLATE SWIRL ICE CREAM: At the start of the fifth hour, spoon ice milk into a freezer container. Stir in ¼ cup Hot Fudgy Milk Chocolate Sauce (page 113). Refreeze until done.

FRUITFUL ICE CREAM: After five hours, when the mixture is still pliable but fairly well frozen, spoon into freezer container. Mix in any sort of chopped fruit you'd like to add. Freeze for another hour.

No-Cook Ice Cream

▼▼▼▼▼▼▼

The previous ice cream recipe produces an ice cream with a puddingy taste. If that doesn't fool your palate well enough, try this recipe, which uses no eggs and requires no cooking. It has a slightly malted taste.

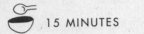 15 MINUTES   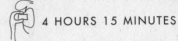 4 HOURS 15 MINUTES

MAKES FOUR ²/₃-CUP SERVINGS.

In a blender, mix:

> **1 cup hot tap water**
> **2 teaspoons powdered gelatin** (1 packet)

Blend on the lowest speed, scraping the sides with a spatula until the gelatin is dissolved.

Add the following ingredients, blending after each addition:

> **²/₃ cup sugar**
> **1 cup skim milk**
> **¹/₃ cup nonfat non-instant dry milk** (available at health food stores)
> **a pinch of salt**
> **1 tablespoon vanilla extract**
> **1 tablespoon lemon juice**

Place blender jar in the freezer. Take out every half hour for 3 hours, scraping the sides and blending on low speed for 30 seconds. Put into a freezer container and freeze another hour.

CHOCOLATE ICE CREAM: Add 4 tablespoons Hot Fudgy Milk Chocolate Sauce (page 113) or 2 tablespoons cocoa powder to the batter. The fat-free serving size is ½ cup.

BANANA ICE CREAM: At the end of the first hour in the freezer, add 2 very ripe sliced bananas when blending.

PEACH ICE CREAM: At the end of the first hour in the freezer, add 1 cup diced fresh or canned peaches.

STRAWBERRY ICE CREAM: At the end of the first hour in the freezer, add 1 cup fresh or thawed frozen strawberries.

HOT FUDGY MILK CHOCOLATE SAUCE

▼▼▼▼▼▼▼

This sauce is quite as thick as a hot fudge sauce. But it keeps its manners whether warm or cold. Its rich puddingy taste and smooth consistency make it a good sauce for cakes, ice cream, and even fruit fondue.

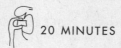 20 MINUTES

MAKES 1 PINT; A 3-TABLESPOON SERVING IS FAT-FREE.

In a medium saucepan, mix:

1½ cups skim milk
½ cup cocoa
1 cup sugar
1 tablespoon arrowroot powder
a pinch of salt
1 teaspoon vanilla extract

Stir over medium-low heat until the sauce starts to thicken, about 10 to 12 minutes. Remove and cool.

Store in the fridge. Shake or stir well before using. The arrowroot gives the sauce enough body that it stands up to heating.

VARIATION: Substitute an equal amount water for the skim milk for a fudge suace that's closer to dark chocolate.

FOR CHOCOLATE FONDUE: Heat up Hot Fudgy Milk Chocolate Sauce and dip banana, apple, and kiwi slices in it, along with strawberries, marshmallows, and squares of Gooey Lemon Cake (page 123). You can also dunk Downy Breadsticks (page 67) in it.

GOOEY CARAMEL SAUCE

▼ ▼ ▼ ▼ ▼ ▼ ▼

Caramel sauce is good atop iced desserts, over cake, and as a dip for apples and other fruits. This recipe can also be made as caramel candy.

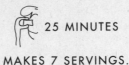 25 MINUTES

MAKES 7 SERVINGS.

In a medium saucepan, mix:

> **1 cup brown sugar**
> **½ cup dark Karo syrup**
> **¼ cup fat-free sour cream**
> **a pinch of salt**

Stir over low heat until the sugar is dissolved. Turn the heat up to medium. When the syrup starts to boil, remove from heat. Let cool 4 minutes. Add:

> **¼ cup fat-free sour cream**

Stir until blended. This sauce is thin enough to be poured when its cool.

FOR A THICKER SAUCE: Add 1 tablespoon cornstarch at the beginning. Good for making caramel apples.

FOR CARAMEL CANDY: Boil syrup mixture until a drop of the syrup forms a cold, soft ball (just slightly softer than a Kraft caramel) when dripped in cold water. Mix in the second ¼ cup of sour cream. While it's cooling for a few minutes, spray a few plastic ice cube trays with vegetable oil cooking spray. You want the caramel to cool enough that it won't melt the ice cube trays. But don't let it cool to the point that it starts to stiffen. Pour into ice cube slots and refrigerate. When the caramels are completely cool, wrap each in wax paper.

Cakes

Cakes can still be rich and moist without fat. I may have gone overboard on cake recipes. But then I could just lose my head over cake. Say, wasn't there a French woman back in the 1700s who . . . never mind.

CREAM-PUFFED CHOCOLATE CUPCAKES

▼ ▼ ▼ ▼ ▼ ▼

Perhaps the world's toughest philosophical question, even more significant than the sound of trees falling or of one hand clapping, is how do they get that filling in those cupcakes? No, they don't bake it in; it would melt. They squirt it in through a tiny hole in the bottom or the top. Disappointing, ain't it?

A similar feat can be duplicated at home in case Bertrand Russell drops by. These cupcakes are also a big hit with kids.

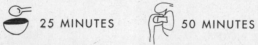 25 MINUTES   50 MINUTES

MAKES 12 SERVINGS.

Preheat oven to **325°F.**

Prepare the batter for **Chocolate Therapy Cake** (page 120).

Lightly coat a muffin tin with cooking spray. Pour the batter in and bake for **25 minutes.**

Let cool and remove from the tin. Using a knife, cut a 1½-inch-deep circle in the top of each cupcake and remove the cupcake "plug." Set aside.

Fill each cupcake with **marshmallow creme.** Carefully replace only the top half inch of the cake "plug."

Ice with Chocolate Buttercream Frosting (page 130), Creamy Caramel Frosting (page 131), or Rich Brownie Frosting (page 131).

Tip: Using Seven-Minute Frosting (pages 128–29) will make this more like a Hostess cupcake but will take about 15 minutes longer.

HEAVY CARROT CAKE

▼ ▼ ▼ ▼ ▼ ▼ ▼

Many fat-free and low-fat cake recipes seem light and empty. This is due to the lack of oil that gives cakes weight. Thanks to the carrots, this cake, on the other hand, is moist and heavy.

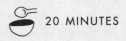 20 MINUTES   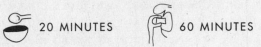 60 MINUTES

MAKES 8 SERVINGS.

Preheat oven to **325°F.**

In a large bowl, mix the following ingredients one at a time. Stir well after each addition:

> **6 egg whites**
> **1½ cup sugar**
> **1 tablespoon vanilla extract**
> **1½ teaspoons ground cinnamon**
> **½ teaspoon ground cloves**
> **½ teaspoon grated nutmeg**
> **3 cups Self-Rising Flour** (page 136; or Health-Rising Flour, page 135)
> **3 cups finely shredded carrots**
> **¾ cup of golden raisins**

Place batter in two 9-inch round cake pans that have been lightly coated with vegetable oil cooking spray and dusted with flour. You can also use a prepared 13 by 9-inch sheet cake pan.

Bake for **35 to 40 minutes.** Cake is done when a toothpick stuck in the center comes out clean.

For a layer cake, let cool 10 minutes. Place a piece of wax paper over one pan. Invert a plate on top of the wax paper. Turn the pan upside down and remove. Turn cake right side up on a cooling rack. Repeat with other pan. Let cool, then frost with Sweet Yogurt Frosting (page 129).

TEXAS SHEET CAKE

▼▼▼▼▼▼▼

Texas Sheet Cake is a cross between brownies and cake. It's iced with chocolate frosting, and it disappears fast.

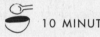 10 MINUTES 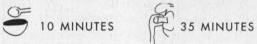 35 MINUTES

MAKES 15 SERVINGS.

Preheat oven to **325°F.**

In a medium bowl, mix the following ingredients one at a time, blending well after each addition:

> ¾ **cup Arrowroot Jelly** (pages 137–38)
> 1½ **cups sugar**
> 3 **egg whites**
> ½ **cup cocoa**
> 1 **tablespoon vanilla extract**
> ½ **teaspoon salt**
> ½ **teaspoon baking powder**
> ¾ **cup flour**

Pour batter into a 13 by 9-inch pan that's been lightly coated with vegetable oil cooking spray and dusted with flour.

Bake for **20 to 25 minutes.**

Let cool. Frost with Rich Brownie Frosting (page 131).

MRS. LOTTIE'S ANGEL FOOD CAKE

▾ ▾ ▾ ▾ ▾ ▾ ▾

Mrs. Lottie doesn't seem a day over twenty. Despite being in her golden years, many a morning she's already cured a ham and crocheted an afghan before the chicken are even thinking about getting up. So in addition to giving you a slice of the finest angel food cake in Nicholas County, Kentucky, she'll sell you a country ham and a cover for your couch. This is a classic recipe that needed no tampering to make it fat-free. (I think she serves it for dessert just to compensate for the fat in the ham.)

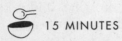 15 MINUTES   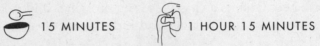 1 HOUR 15 MINUTES

MAKES 8 OVERWHELMING FAT-FREE SERVINGS.

Preheat oven to **350° F.** (Mrs. Lottie's recipe says 325° F., but that's only if you're using an old gas oven.)

In a large bowl, place:

>   **2 cups egg whites plus 2 egg whites** (about 13 total)
>   **1 teaspoon cream of tartar**

Whip with an electric mixer until the egg whites form stiff peaks. Using a wire whisk, GENTLY stir in:

>   **2 cups Swan's Down cake flour** (that's been sifted 4 times)
>   **3 cups sugar**
>   **½ teaspoon salt**
>   **1 teaspoon vanilla extract**

Pour into an angel food cake pan or Bundt pan.

Bake for **45 minutes.**

Turn off the oven and let the cake sit in there for **15 minutes** to brown. Turn the pan upside down over a cake plate. Cover with a damp cloth to help loosen the cake. Let sit for 1 hour, then remove cake from pan.

VARIATION: Any kind of extract can be used. Double the amount to 2 teaspoons, if you like.

MOIST JAM CAKE
▼▼▼▼▼▼▼

Jam cake is a traditional favorite. The oil is missing but not missed, since the jam keeps the cake moist. The traditional jam to use in this recipe is blackberry, but any kind of jam or preserve works. If you think blackberry seeds are too gritty, try strawberry preserves.

 15 MINUTES 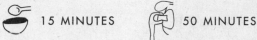 50 MINUTES

MAKES 12 SERVINGS.

Preheat oven to **350°F.**

In a large bowl, mix the following ingredients one at a time, stirring well after each addition:

1½ cups sugar
½ cup buttermilk
5 egg whites
2¼ cups flour
1 teaspoon ground allspice
1 teaspoon ground cinnamon
1 teaspoon grated nutmeg
½ teaspoon salt
1 teaspoon baking powder
½ teaspoon baking soda
1 cup jam

Pour batter into a 13 by 9-inch cake pan that's been lightly coated with vegetable oil cooking spray and dusted with flour.

Bake for **35 minutes,** or until a toothpick comes out clean when you stick it in the middle of the cake.

When cool, frost with Creamy Caramel Frosting (page 131).

CHOCOLATE THERAPY CAKE

▾ ▾ ▾ ▾ ▾ ▾ ▾

This is an excellent bad-water, drown-your-sorrows, woe-is-me, my-lover-ran-off-with-a-Home-Shopping-Network-pitch-person kind of cake.

It's rich and chocolaty and always forces you to eat one more piece. Go ahead, have a nice big fat-free slice.

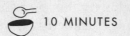 10 MINUTES   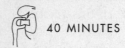 40 MINUTES

MAKES 10 SERVINGS.

Preheat oven to **325°F.**

In a medium bowl, mix the following ingredients one at a time, stirring well after each addition:

> **6 egg whites**
> **¾ cup sugar**
> **1 tablespoon vanilla extract**
> **¾ cup flour**
> **⅓ cup cocoa**
> **½ teaspoon salt**
> **1 teaspoon baking powder**
> **1½ cups marshmallow creme**

Mix until the marshmallow lumps are gone. Pour batter into a 9 by 9-inch pan that's been lightly coated with vegetable oil cooking spray.

Bake for **30 minutes.**

You can eat the cake warm from the oven. It goes well with a glass of milk. It's also good dipped *in* the glass of milk. For really depressing times, or around tax season, submerge a piece of cake in Hot Fudgy Milk Chocolate Sauce (page 113).

GOOEY COCOA CAKE

▼▼▼▼▼▼

This cakes tastes homemade. It's moist and rich, and slightly heavier than a cake-mix cake. It's like the cake that nice old lady down the street used to bring over before they carted her away for securities fraud.

Though the applesauce is undetectable, it keeps the cake moist. Eat it plain, or sprinkled with powdered sugar, or smothered with syrup. This recipe is for a 9 by 9-inch sheet cake. If you double it, you'll get a little more batter than you'll need for two round layer cakes.

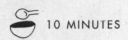 10 MINUTES   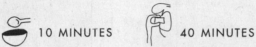 40 MINUTES

MAKES 10 SERVINGS.

Preheat oven to **350° F.**

Mix in the follow ingredients one at a time, stirring well after each addition:

> **2 egg whites**
> **1 cup sugar**
> **1 cup flour**
> **⅓ cup cocoa**
> **½ cup applesauce**
> **½ teaspoon salt**
> **1 teaspoon vanilla extract**
> **1 teaspoon baking soda**
> **1 tablespoon lemon juice**

Pour batter into a 9 by 9-inch nonstick baking pan that's been lightly coated with vegetable oil cooking spray and dusted with flour.

Bake for **30 minutes.**

Note: The batter can also be poured into a muffin tin for chocolate muffins. Bake for 15 minutes.

GOOEY SPICE CAKE

▼ ▼ ▼ ▼ ▼ ▼

Another moist, homemade-tasting cake. It's a good recipe to try on people who say that fat-free desserts taste awful. Never tell them, just smile when they ask.

This recipe is for a 9 by 9-inch sheet cake. If you double it, you'll get a little more batter than you'll need for two round layer cakes.

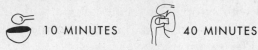

10 MINUTES   40 MINUTES

MAKES 5 SERVINGS.

Preheat oven to **350°F.**

Mix in the follow ingredients one at a time, stirring well after each addition:

> **2 egg whites**
> **1 cup sugar**
> **1¼ cups flour**
> **½ cup applesauce**
> **½ teaspoon salt**
> **1 teaspoon vanilla extract**
> **1 teaspoon baking soda**
> **1 teaspoon ground cinnamon**
> **¼ teaspoon ground cloves**
> **¼ teaspoon ground allspice**
> **¼ teaspoon grated nutmeg**
> **a pinch of ground ginger**
> **1 tablespoon lemon juice**

Pour batter into a 9 by 9-inch nonstick baking pan that's been lightly coated with vegetable oil cooking spray and dusted with flour. Bake for **30 minutes.**

Ice with Seven-Minute Frosting (pages 128–29), Creamy Caramel Frosting (page 131), Buttercream Frosting (page 127), or even Chocolate Buttercream Frosting (page 130).

Note: You can also bake in a muffin tin for 15 minutes.

Gooey Lemon Cake

▼▼▼▼▼▼

Lemon cake is especially good in the summer. This one will bring back memories of family reunions and sitting in front of the TV after dinner watching the Roadrunner get the best of Wile E. Coyote. It's a moist cake that's heavier than a box cake, but lighter than a Bundt cake. There's applesauce in it, but you can't taste it.

This recipe is for a 9 by 9-inch sheet cake. But it rises fairly high, just about enough to fill two round layer cake pans.

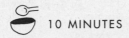 10 MINUTES 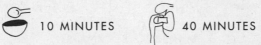 40 MINUTES

MAKES 5 SERVINGS.

Preheat your oven to **350°F.**

Mix in the following ingredients one at a time, stirring well after each addition:

> **2 egg whites**
> **1 cup sugar**
> **1½ cups flour**
> **½ cup applesauce**
> **½ teaspoon salt**
> **1 teaspoon vanilla extract**
> **1 teaspoon baking soda**
> **½ teaspoon ground cardamom** (optional)
> **½ teaspoon ground coriander** (optional)
> **¼ cup lemon juice**
> **2 tablespoons fresh grated lemon zest**

Pour batter into a 9 by 9-inch nonstick baking pan that's been lightly coated with vegetable oil cooking spray and dusted with flour.

Bake for **30 minutes.** Ice with lemon buttercream frosting (page 127) or eat plain.

Note: You can also bake in a muffin tin for 15 minutes.

WHITE MIRACLE CAKE

▼ ▼ ▼ ▼ ▼ ▼ ▼

A good layer cake recipe is the most useful cake recipe you can have. Miracle cake can be used for double- or triple-layer birthday cakes and sheet cakes. It can be flavored with extracts and tinted with food coloring. It doesn't rise as high as boxed mix, but it's very moist and spongy.

This recipe is based on an Amish recipe that uses Miracle Whip instead of oil.

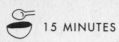 15 MINUTES   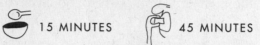 45 MINUTES

MAKES 22 SERVINGS.

BUT BE CAREFUL: ¹/₂₂ OF THE CAKE IS ESTIMATED TO CONTAIN ONE-HALF GRAM OF FAT. (KRAFT IS RELUCTANT TO GIVE THE EXACT FAT CONTENT OF THEIR FAT-FREE MIRACLE WHIP.) THIS CAKE RECIPE IS VERY FLEXIBLE. TRY ANY OF THE VARIATIONS.

Preheat oven to **375°F.**

In a large bowl, put:

> **1 cup fat-free Miracle Whip**
> **1 cup warm water**

Beat until light. Add the following ingredients, mixing well after each:

> **1 cup sugar**
> **1 teaspoon vanilla extract**
> **¼ teaspoon salt**
> **2 teaspoons baking soda**
> **2 cups cake flour**

Pour into two 8-inch or 9-inch round nonstick cake pans that have been sprayed with vegetable oil cooking spray and dusted with flour. A 13 by 9-inch sheet cake pan can also be used.

Bake for **32 minutes.** A toothpick should come out clean when stuck in the cake. For layer cake pans, cool 10 minutes. Put a piece of wax paper on top of the cake. Invert a plate on top of the wax paper. Turn over. The cake should fall right out. Place right side up on cooling rack. Repeat with other layer. When cool, stack the layers and ice with Buttercream Frosting (page 127).

SPICE CAKE: Add ½ teaspoon ground cloves, ¼ teaspoon ground allspice, ½ teaspoon grated nutmeg, and 1½ teaspoons ground cinnamon to the batter. You can also add ½ cup dates or golden raisins.

ALMOND CAKE: Add 1 teaspoon almond extract.

LEMON CAKE: Add 1 teaspoon lemon extract and 1 tablespoon fresh grated lemon zest.

ORANGE CAKE: Add 1 teaspoon orange extract and 1 tablespoon fresh grated orange zest.

EXTRACTS VS. FLAVORINGS

The recipes in this book call for extracts to be used whenever possible. Extracts are essences that have been extracted from a natural source, such as vanilla or lemons. They are extracted with alcohol or oil. It's best to use alcohol-based extracts. The alcohol evaporates during cooking. Essential oils are potent condensed extracts. Where you would use a teaspoon of extract, three drops of an essential oil are all that's needed.

Flavorings are usually synthetic substances that mimic the taste of an extract. They almost never come close to the original. They are cheaper than extracts, but for the best taste, stick to the real thing.

CHOCOLATE MIRACLE CAKE

▼▼▼▼▼▼

This is a good moist chocolate cake.

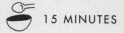 15 MINUTES   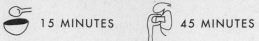 45 MINUTES

MAKES 27 SERVINGS.

BUT BE CAREFUL: $1/27$ OF THE CAKE CONTAINS LESS THAN $1/2$ GRAM OF FAT. THE ACTUAL FAT-FREE PORTION IS PROBABLY LARGER, BUT KRAFT REFUSES TO GIVE THE EXACT FAT CONTENT OF THEIR FAT-FREE MIRACLE WHIP.

Preheat oven to **375°F.**

In a large bowl, put:

> **1 cup fat-free Miracle Whip**
> **1 cup warm water**

Beat until light. Add the following ingredients, mixing well after each:

> **1 cup sugar**
> **4 tablespoons cocoa**
> **1 teaspoon vanilla extract**
> **¼ teaspoon salt**
> **2 teaspoons baking soda**
> **2 cups cake flour**

Pour into two 8-inch or 9-inch round cake pans that have been sprayed with vegetable oil cooking spray and dusted with flour. A 13 by 9-inch sheet cake pan can also be used.

Bake for **32 minutes.** A toothpick should come out clean when stuck in the cake.

For layer cake pans, cool 10 minutes. Put a piece of wax paper on top of the cake. Invert a plate on top of the wax paper. Turn over. The cake should fall right out. Place right side up on the cooling rack. Repeat with other cake. When cool, ice with Chocolate Buttercream Frosting (page 130).

MOCHA CAKE: Replace warm water with 1 cup warm coffee.

CHOCOLATE VELVET CAKE: Add 2 teaspoons red food coloring. (Some people also add 1 teaspoon of non-oil-based cherry extract.) Ice with Buttercream Frosting (below) or Seven-Minute Frosting (pages 128–29). You can also put maraschino cherry halves on top. They're fat-free.

BUTTERCREAM FROSTING

▼▼▼▼▼▼▼

Thanks to fat-free margarine, nonfat buttercream frosting is now possible. However, some people find that fat-free margarine, in addition to having a synthetic texture, has a chemical taste. If you've tried the margarine and you think the taste is odd, you're better off going with another frosting recipe.

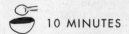 10 MINUTES

MAKES 1 CUP; ENOUGH FROSTING TO COVER ⅛ OF THE CAKE IS FAT-FREE.

Place **¼ cup soft-spread fat-free margarine** in a medium mixing bowl.

Slowly add **2 cups powdered sugar,** stirring well after each addition.

Stir in **1 teaspoon vanilla extract.** The frosting is ready to be spread onto the cake.

For best results, store the frosted cake in the refrigerator.

VARIATION: In place of the vanilla extract, try almond extract, lemon extract, or mint extract. The frosting can also be tinted with food coloring.

SEVEN-MINUTE FROSTING

▼ ▼ ▼ ▼ ▼ ▼ ▼

Whipped cream is sorely missed by those trying to cut back on their fat intake. Even a small amount of the real thing is deadly, containing up to forty-four grams of fat per cup. Go ahead, it's okay to gasp. Even nondairy toppings contain one gram of fat—in a measly tablespoon. Seven-Minute Frosting, on the other hand, contains no fat in an entire batch.

This frosting dries out quickly, so keep whatever you put it on refrigerated. In addition to cake, it's also good for frosting brownies and cookies and filling cookie sandwiches.

 20 MINUTES

MAKES 12 SERVINGS.

In a medium saucepan, place:

2 egg whites
¼ teaspoon cream of tartar (optional)
1 cup sugar
1 tablespoon light Karo syrup

Mix well. Add:

1 tablespoon water
a pinch of salt

Cook over low heat, whipping regularly with a wire whisk. Remove from heat when the frosting forms soft peaks. (When you pull out the whisk, the mountains will rise and the peaks will fall.)

Stir in:

1 tablespoon vanilla extract

Spread onto cake before the frosting cools.

VARIATIONS: This is a fairly flexible recipe. In place of the vanilla you can add 1 tablespoon instant coffee granules; 1 tablespoon grated lemon, orange, or lime zest; or 3 drops essential peppermint oil. Caramel frosting can be made by substituting ⅔ cup brown sugar for the white sugar.

SWEET YOGURT FROSTING
▼ ▼ ▼ ▼ ▼ ▼ ▼

This is a slightly more exotic twist on cream cheese frosting. It's both sweeter and tarter.

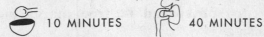 10 MINUTES   40 MINUTES

MAKES 1½ CUPS;
THE ENTIRE BATCH OF FROSTING IS FAT-FREE.

Put:

> ½ **cup nonfat yogurt** in a handkerchief or a square of cheesecloth.

Gather the ends and tie them around a spoon handle. Dangle the yogurt over a bowl using the spoon handle to suspend it. Let sit about 40 minutes. Gently twist until the handkerchief tightens around the ball of yogurt. More liquid should drip out. Don't twist so hard that the yogurt oozes out. Put the yogurt in a medium bowl.

Add:

> **1 teaspoon vanilla extract**
> **1 tablespoon fresh lemon juice**
> **3 cups powdered sugar**

Blend until smooth. Spread on cake. To keep the frosting from running, keep the cake refrigerated.

CHOCOLATE BUTTERCREAM FROSTING

▼▼▼▼▼▼▼

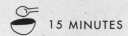

15 MINUTES

MAKES ENOUGH TO ICE A 13 BY 9-INCH SHEET CAKE OR TWO 9-INCH SINGLE-LAYER CAKES; EACH TABLESPOON OF FROSTING IS FAT-FREE.

Place **¼ cup soft-spread fat-free margarine** into a medium mixing bowl.

Add **4 tablespoons cocoa.** Mix well.

Slowly add **2 cups powdered sugar,** mixing well after each addition.

Beat in **1 teaspoon vanilla extract.** For a darker frosting, add 7 drops red and 2 drops green food coloring.

SEPARATING EGG WHITES

There's an art to separating the white without breaking the yolk. Commercial separator cups with slit sides are available, but not necessary.

1. Crack the egg on a sharp surface with a quick, light blow. This keeps the shell from shattering. Next, with the egg upright, pull the top straight off.

2. Over a bowl, gently pour the yolk back and forth between the halves. The white will pour out, and the yolk will be left intact. For what to do with your egg yolks, see page 138.

CREAMY CARAMEL FROSTING

▼▼▼▼▼▼▼

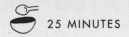 25 MINUTES 25 MINUTES

MAKES 1 CUP; FROSTING FOR HALF THE CAKE IS FAT-FREE.

In a medium saucepan, mix:

2 cups brown sugar
½ cup buttermilk

Boil over medium heat, stirring constantly. With your cooking spoon, drip a few drops of the boiling liquid into a cup of cold water. When you can pick these droplets up with your fingers, the frosting is done. Remove from heat. Let it cool for 10 minutes. Beat until it starts to stiffen and lightens in color. Immediately spread the frosting on a cooled cake.

RICH BROWNIE FROSTING

▼▼▼▼▼▼▼

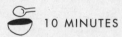 10 MINUTES

MAKES ENOUGH TO ICE 13 BY 9-INCH SHEET CAKE.
ONE-THIRD OF THE BATCH CONTAINS LESS THAN ONE-HALF
GRAM OF FAT.

Mix in the following ingredients one at a time, stirring well after each addition:

3 tablespoons Arrowroot Jelly (pages 137–38)
3 tablespoons cocoa
1 tablespoon corn syrup
1 teaspoon vanilla extract
2 tablespoons skim milk
1 cup powdered sugar

Don't think drinks are fattening? Look at the back of that eggnog carton. Ask your bartender how much butter is in that rum. These fat-free beverages are rich and tasty enough to skip dessert.

BANANA EGGNOG

▼ ▼ ▼ ▼ ▼ ▼ ▼

This is a surprisingly versatile recipe. You can use it to make thick eggnog, eggnog pudding, or eggnog ice milk.

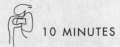 10 MINUTES

MAKES 5 SERVINGS.

In a 2-quart saucepan, mix:

> **12 ounces Egg Beaters**
> **2 to 3 overly ripe bananas** (puréed)
> **⅓ cup sugar**
> **3 cups skim milk**
> **a pinch of ground cloves**
> **¼ teaspoon grated nutmeg**
> **1 tablespoon nonfat non-instant dry milk**
>   (available at health food stores)
> **1 teaspoon rum extract**

Cook over medium-low heat until it's as thick as you want it.

VARIATION: Spike with ½ cup dark rum or whiskey.

BANANA NOG PUDDING: Add 1 tablespoon cornstarch. Cook over medium-low heat until thick. Spoon into serving dishes and dash with nutmeg.

BANANA NOG ICE CREAM: Cook over medium-low heat until thick. Put into blender. Freeze in the blender jar for 5 hours. Take out every hour to scrape the sides of the jar and blend on low for 30 seconds. Spoon into serving dishes. Top with Gooey Caramel Sauce (page 114).

HOT SPICED CIDER

▼ ▼ ▼ ▼ ▼ ▼ ▼

This recipe should be part of any winter survival kit. It's especially good if you have some fresh cider that's starting to go hard.

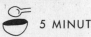 5 MINUTES   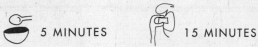 15 MINUTES

MAKES 4 SERVINGS.

In a medium saucepan, mix:

4 cups apple cider
2 tablespoons honey
1 teaspoon ground cinnamon
a pinch of ground cloves

Simmer 10 minutes and serve hot.

VARIATION: Spike each cup with 2 tablespoons dark rum. Cranapple juice can be substituted for the cider.

GAINBACK

There's a very successful company that has diet centers throughout the country. You see their ads all the time. You buy their food. The pounds melt away. HOWEVER: Their own estimates show that 90 percent of their clients gain it all back—plus some extra!

The body is very unforgiving to those who have lost weight. If you go back to eating like you used to, you will gain even faster than you did before. The body tries to stockpile fat in an effort to recoup its former stores.

The only successful way to keep weight off is to adapt permanent healthy eating habits.

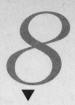

Substitutions

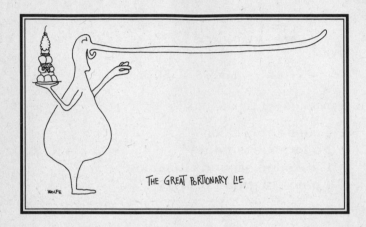

THE GREAT PORTIONARY LIE

- ▶ **HEALTH-RISING FLOUR**
- ▶ **SELF-RISING FLOUR**
- ▶ **BUTTERMILK**
- ▶ **ARROWROOT JELLY**

As a rule, substitutions aren't recommended. Many of the recipes in this book require precise measurements to get them to work correctly. If one ingredient is altered, the recipe fails.

Fresh, natural ingredients are always recommended, because imitation flavorings seldom taste as good as the real thing. The following substitutions can be made, but the final product may not turn out exactly the same.

HEALTH-RISING FLOUR
▼ ▼ ▼ ▼ ▼ ▼ ▼

Most commercially made self-rising flours use baking powder that contains aluminum. If this is a health concern for you, this recipe for Health-Rising Flour uses an aluminum-free baking powder. This flour can be substituted cup for cup in place of self-rising flour. The whole wheat flour makes breads weightier. They won't rise as much, but they take on a heartier, more wholesome flavor.

The following recipe is for each cup of self-rising flour needed. For convenience, mix up a larger batch and store in a flour container.

Or mix:

$\frac{1}{2}$ **cup unbleached white flour**
$\frac{1}{2}$ **cup whole wheat pastry flour** (available at most health food stores)
$1\frac{1}{2}$ **teaspoons Rumford baking powder** (available at health food stores and grocery stores)
$\frac{1}{2}$ **teaspoon sea salt**

SELF-RISING FLOUR

▼▼▼▼▼▼▼

Mix the quantity needed in the following proportions:

**1 cup flour
1 teaspoon baking powder
½ teaspoon salt**

BUTTERMILK

▼▼▼▼▼▼▼

Most people don't keep buttermilk on hand. These recipes should work in a pinch. They make the equivalent of one cup of buttermilk. The skim milk also slightly reduces the fat content of any buttermilk recipe.

Mix:

**1 cup skim milk
2 tablespoons white vinegar**

Or mix:

**1 cup skim milk
4 tablespoons buttermilk powder**

Allow to sit **20 minutes.** Stir before using.

CARBOHYDRATE WEIGHT

Notice how you can gain or lose four pounds in a day, then the next day lose or gain it back again? For years cheap bathroom scales were blamed. But the true culprit may be carbohydrate weight.

We used to think all carbohydrates (starches and sugars) go to fat. But on a normal day only one twentieth of your carbohydrate intake goes to fat. All of your daily fat intake above forty grams or so, on the other hand, can go to fat.

Your liver and muscles store a small amount of excess carbohydrates and a lot of water along with them. It's possible to retain six pounds of water with carbohydrates. The good news is that within a few days, excess carbohydrates burn off and you lose the water weight along with them.

Egg Beaters and Egg Substitutes

Only a few recipes in this book call for Egg Beaters. They're expensive, so many people opt to use the same amount of plain egg whites instead. The only reason that Egg Beaters are used in Banana Eggnog (pages 132–133) and La Toast Française (page 44) is because they add color. If you use egg whites in a recipe and still want yellow color, you can use yellow food coloring or a pinch of turmeric, a spice available at most larger grocery stores. (Use no more than a pinch, though, or you'll change the flavor.) Another natural option is beta-carotene, found in carrots. One-half teaspoon of fresh carrot juice (not canned) will give a warmer color but won't change the flavor.

ARROWROOT JELLY

▼ ▼ ▼ ▼ ▼ ▼ ▼

One of the most valuable fat-cutting recipes is one that you'll never eat by itself. Arrowroot Jelly is a flavorless, clear, fat-free starch jelly that replaces oil in many recipes. If you substitute an equal amount of Arrowroot Jelly for oil in a salad dressing mix, the dressing will have a similar taste, texture, and appearance. Arrowroot Jelly bakes lighter than oil, but the end product looks like it was baked with oil. The jelly also adds body and smoothness to frozen desserts.

Arrowroot powder is finer than cornstarch and makes a much smoother jelly. If you have no arrowroot powder, you can substitute cornstarch, but it won't be quite as smooth. Buy arrowroot powder at a health food store. If you buy it at your corner grocery, an ounce or two can cost up to three dollars. If you buy it bulk-packed at the health food store, a pint container can be as cheap as a dollar.

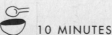 10 MINUTES

In a saucepan, place:

3 tablespoons arrowroot powder

Slowly add:

1 cup water

Mix until smooth. Stir over high heat until the jelly boils and clears. Remove from heat. Use after cooling a few minutes, or store in the fridge for up to two weeks. If it starts to separate after a week or so, boil again.

WHAT TO DO WITH YOUR EGG YOLKS

Many of the recipes in this book call for egg whites; Mrs. Lottie's Angel Food Cake calls for thirteen. That leaves you with a lot of yolks.

Yolks contain almost six grams of fat each, so for our purposes of fat-free cooking, they've been left out. But don't throw them away. There are many things you can do with egg yolks.

1. Organize an egg yolk exchange. Many German, Hungarian, and Middle European cooks use only egg yolks and throw out their egg whites. Store your yolks in zipper bags in the freezer, with a dozen in each bag.

2. Blend them with latex for a beautiful yellow paint. Note, however, that the room may take on the smell of sulfur.

3. Get back at the kids who squirt you with squirt guns. Two dozen yolks fill a super-soaker quite nicely.

4. Throw at politicians, provided this is an accepted practice in your area.

5. On days when the door-to-door salespeople come calling, smear yolk on your doorbell button. I don't know if it's the sight of the bright ooze that keeps them away or it could be that they're superstitious about the color yellow.

6. Age yolks properly and mail them to Third World tyrants.

INDEX

INDEX

CONVERSION CHART

Equivalent Imperial and Metric Measurements

American cooks use standard containers, the 8-ounce cup and a tablespoon that takes exactly 16 level fillings to fill that cup level. Measuring by cup makes it very difficult to give weight equivalents, as a cup of densely packed butter will weigh considerably more than a cup of flour. The easiest way therefore to deal with cup measurements in recipes is to take the amount by volume rather than by weight. Thus the equation reads:

$$1 \text{ cup} = 240 \text{ ml} = 8 \text{ fl. oz.} \quad \tfrac{1}{2} \text{ cup} = 120 \text{ ml} = 4 \text{ fl. oz.}$$

It is possible to buy a set of American cup measures in major stores around the world. In the States, butter is often measured in sticks. One stick is the equivalent of 8 tablespoons. One tablespoon of butter is therefore the equivalent to ½ ounce/15 grams.

Liquid Measures

Fluid ounces	U.S.	Imperial	Milliliters
	1 tsp	1 tsp	5
¼	2 tsps	1 dessertspoon	10
½	1 tbs	1 tbs	14
1	2 tbs	2 tbs	28
2	¼ cup	4 tbs	56
4	½ cup		110
5		¼ pint or 1 gill	140
6	¾ cup		170
8	1 cup		225
9			250, ¼ liter
10	1¼ cups	½ pint	280
12	1½ cups		340
15		¾ pint	420
16	2 cups		450
18	2¼ cups		500, ½ liter
20	2½ cups	1 pint	560
24	3 cups		675
25		1¼ pints	700
27	3½ cups		750
30	3¾ cups	1½ pints	840
32	4 cups or 1 quart		900

Solid Measures

U.S. and Imperial Measures ounces	pounds	Metric Measures grams	kilos
1		28	
2		56	
3½		100	
4	¼	112	
5		140	
6		168	
8	½	225	
9		250	¼
12	¾	340	
16	1	450	
18		500	½

Oven Temperature Equivalents

Farenheit	Celsius	Gas Mark	Description
225	110	¼	Cool
275	140	1	Very Slow
325	170	3	Slow
350	180	4	Moderate
400	200	6	Moderately Hot
425	220	7	Fairly Hot
450	230	8	Hot
500	250	10	Extremely Hot